Praise for *Reimagining Women's Self-Defense*

"A close friend paid her way through college by working as a stripper. She hired me to bodyguard her and her fellow performers whenever they did private shows. To be clear, they were not sex workers, but some clients wouldn't take 'no' for an answer without my intervention. I soon discovered that job wasn't the only reason she had to view the world around her differently than I did. Our conversations were thought-provoking, highlighting a variety of subjects that I have rarely seen in woman's self-defense prior to reading this book. Let's face it, most martial arts were designed by men, primarily for men, hence fail to account for differences in biology, threat vectors, and lifestyle. *Reimagining Woman's Self-Defense* corrects traditional misconceptions, advocating a framework of protective offense with proven strategies for avoiding danger, de-escalating conflict, and fighting back effectively. It's well-written, practical, and an important call to action that should be embraced by anyone who wants to help women move through the world more safely."

—**Lawrence Kane**, Sensei, American Martial Arts Alliance (AMAA) Who's Who in the Martial Arts Hall of Honors Inductee, SIG Sourcing Supernova Hall of Fame Member, ProcureCon EPIC Lifetime Achievement Award Winner, bestselling multi-award-winning author of thirty-one books, including *Musashi's Dokkodo, The Little Black Book of Violence, The Big Bloody Book of Violence, How to Win a Fight,* and *Surviving Armed Assaults*

"*Reimagining Women's Self-Defense* shatters the centuries-old beliefs of women in conflict then reshapes them to strengthen every weapon in the arsenal for optimum mental, emotional, and physical self-defense. Teja VanWicklen's expertise, personal story, and life-long passion for the fighting arts have culminated in this brilliant book, one that is certain to advance and elevate women's training for years to come."

—**Lori Hartman Gervasi**, author of *Fight Like a Girl...and Win: Defense Decisions for Women*

"Women face unique situations and challenges, yet most traditional martial arts training fails to address them adequately or does so only in the most general terms. Teja VanWicklen's *Reimagining Women's Self-Defense* seeks to fill that gap and does so admirably, drawing on her many years of training and personal experiences growing up in the heart of New York City. With compelling stories, raw honesty, and hard-won wisdom, Teja dispenses genuinely useful, pragmatic advice that applies to real-world situations, much of which I have never heard discussed in any martial arts class. Teja has boldly reimagined women's self-defense beyond mere fighting techniques: she considers lifestyle, psychology (of both criminals and their intended victims), situational awareness, trauma recovery, health and nutrition, legal concerns, and more—because truly effective self-defense doesn't happen in the vacuum of traditional martial arts training."

—**Jennifer Ouellette**, author of *Me Myself, and Why,* science journalist, recipient of science writing award (Acoustical Society of America), 2018 Humanist of the Year (American Humanist Association), Shodan Niseido Jujitsu

"I have been a single parent since my kids were six months old. I was in deployment-ready units until the oldest went to university and have several missions and exercises, domestic and international, while parenting very young children. The challenges working single parents face are already monumental, then add to them the threat of physical violence. I felt genuine fear taking them out alone in certain areas. Fortunately for me, Teja and I were both looking for ways to better ourselves. She happened to be giving a class on women's self-defense (not a traditional one), and I immediately signed up. The course was eye-opening and life changing. Teja spelled out in simple terms why traditional 'self-defense' courses fell short of the mark, leaving many with a false sense of security.

"I was immediately drawn to her way of speaking about women's self-defense. Teja spoke a language I understood, and even though we were both physically very strong and capable women, the reality of infants and toddlers brought a world of problems which, even with with my skillset, I felt completely unprepared for. I had completed difficult training in Army combat trades; I'd learned loads about how to survive in the wild, how to take care of equipment, and how to move safely in various environments or inclement weather. I had taken intense first-aid for deployments. Yet I was unsure of how to confront a dangerous situation with a stroller, a diaper bag, and a toddler or two in tow. After having had to chase three on a beach, all at once, in three separate and equally dangerous directions (road, nettle patch, and water) with a compromised bikini top, it was clear I needed to up my safety game.

"I encourage all women who suddenly find themselves on uneven footing as new parents to read this book. I am so grateful for Teja and her work and firmly believe we can all benefit from her knowledge. It takes a village, and she has my vote for Chief."
—**Sgt Deloris Del Rio**, CD (ret.)

"As a wheelchair user and founder of a self-defense instruction nonprofit, I have reached the same conclusion as Teja regarding the state of self-defense for women—it is badly in need of a makeover.

"*Reimaging Women's Self-Defense* is a strategic plan of action for women. [It is] loaded with personal stories and references to relevant subject matter and arms women and self-defense instructors with a clear and concise instructional framework.

"The self-defense industry is both male-dominated and fighting-centric; the 'self-defense' aspect is more defense of ego than anything else. *Reimaging Women's Self-Defense* is a deep dive into personal protection. It is the culmination of Teja's many years of intense study and well worth your time."

—**Erik Kondo**, 3rd degree black belt in Small Circle Jujitsu, founder of self-defense nonprofit *NOT-ME! Inc.*, author of *Not-Me! Self-Defense and the Martial Arts for and by People with SCI/D*

"*Reimagining Women's Self-Defense* came to me at exactly the right time in my life. Pre-pandemic I [was an instructor with] Street Sheild Self-Defense—I taught the soft skills and performed demonstrations while my sensei taught the physical skills. Since then, I've suffered a series of serious injuries that have left me wondering what I can still contribute to teaching.

"Teja's book made me think deeply and productively. I learned not only from her own experiences but also from the brilliant way she organized the book using the Self-Defense Continuum. This reminded me that the soft skills are actually the most important part of any women's self-defense training.

"Teja's experience in life and on the mat puts her in the forefront of teaching the people who actually need it: women, injured women, women who must protect others. My children are grown so I protect my elderly mom. Teja is centering and naming that truth."

—**Amy Stewart-Cooper**, ADHD Leadership Coach, 500 Rising Endorsed Colleague, co-instructor Street Shield Self-Defense, 2nd degree black belt (Nidan) Okinawan Kenpo

"Teja's journey as a female practitioner in martial arts will resonate with other women who have confronted the outlier experience of being the only woman on the mat. Her writing begins with what it means to be a female practitioner 'screaming into the void' of combat fighting systems designed by and for men. If you too are one of those women—you will feel heard in these pages.

"For the adventurous martial arts novice, the material will help guide your training in what is still a male-oriented profession (in approach, technique, and curriculum). The information in these pages ranges from critical prevention skills to Teja's recommendations for foundational physical responses to the last threshold in self-defense—the physical fight. For the coach, trainer, and seasoned practitioner, Teja has accomplished a Herculean challenge, organizing mountains of information into chapters and closing with bulleted summaries and applicable exercises whether or not you are training with a dojo. As the book concludes, she tells the reader, 'The best way to learn anything is to use it.' Throughout each chapter, she provides suggestions on how to do exactly that. Enjoy!"

—**Tammy Yard-McCracken**, PsyD, LPC., krav maga instructor, certified Conflict Communication instructor, self-defense instructor, founder of Kore Self-Defense & Krav Maga, violence dynamics instructor, founder and CEO 500Rising, Inc., speaker, corporate trainer, and psychotherapist with experience in trauma recovery and survivors of violence

"As a physical educator, martial-arts practitioner and instructor, and security professional, I have found that the more I train and study self-defense and survival arts, the more I understand the importance of learning the most realistic, current, and practical skills from top instructors and reputable sources. However, physical skill is only a small part of the equation. *Reimagining Women's Self-Defense* offers a comprehensive, well-researched, and thought-provoking overview of broader knowledge. To that end, the author incorporated personal anecdotes, relevant quotes, acronyms, and sketches throughout the text. She also integrated devices created by renowned experts into the 'Self-Defense Continuum,' a model that clearly outlines the complex process of crime in a format that is easy for the average person to understand. This manuscript is an essential read for anyone seeking to gain the mental, emotional, and physical tools to protect themselves and loved ones from violent threats if necessary. Knowledge is power, and a well-informed, tactical mindset is the ultimate weapon. This book provides... and then some!"

—**Rick Mitchell**, 4th-degree black belt Modern Arnis, fully qualified instructor Taboada Balintawak Escrima, International World Cup Full-Contact Stick Fighting Grand Champion, Pan-American Brazilian Jujitsu Champion, security professional

"Holistic, informative, and intelligent. This is a book that has been needed for quite some time. I read it with some expectation, having seen some of the author's work before, and it did not disappoint.

"It is not a rehash but rather a serious look at what is needed for good, effective self-defense, filtered to be more accessible and applicable to women and other marginalized people and communities. It does not rely on fear to sell its lessons; it relies on knowledge, facts, and personal experience. What's more, it closes out each section with action points that teach you to integrate what you have just learned into your life, internally, not as a costume.

"Teja includes all of the various aspects I think are required to take care of oneself in the modern environment, including the use of effective weapons, and she even gets into some first aid in the aftermath of a critical incident.

"I am glad to see this book come out, and highly recommend it to everyone, especially women—it is needed."

—**Terry Trahan**, Senior Instructor Aneh Palu Kali-Silat, Director of the Kapatiran Suntukan Martial Arts Organization, protection specialist, bouncer

"Recently, a female student asked me which martial art would be best for self-defense. I answered her truthfully: none. There is a small amount of self-defense knowledge that can be extracted from martial arts.

"In *Reimagining Women's Self Defense,* Teja has drawn on her extensive experience, synthesized some excellent material, and sourced knowledge from experts in their respective fields to provide a unique resource for women seeking self-defense guidance. I will be recommending this book to the women, and men, who train with me here in the United Kingdom."

—**Garry Smith,** 5th Dan Black Belt in traditional Jujitsu (British Combat Association); Chief Instructor at the Academy of Self-Defense, UK; Post Graduate Degree in Educational Management

"Too many self-defense resources are offered by large, athletic men with law enforcement or military experience. Although I have immense respect for those men, they know very little about the safety of women. How could they? Their size, experience, relationship with violence, and even the sort of predator who might attack them are entirely different from what a soccer mom, college co-ed, or business executive might face.

"Teja VanWicklen does more than identify this problem. She presents solutions in a scientifically grounded, street-tested, and above all usable framework that can be applied today. Women, parents of girls, and every martial artist or self-defense instructor should read this book."

—**Jason Brick,** 6th-degree black belt in Kenpo, host of the podcast "Safest Family on the Block," author of *Safest Family on the Block,* and *There I Was…When Nothing Happened*

REIMAGINING WOMEN'S SELF-DEFENSE

REIMAGINING WOMEN'S SELF-DEFENSE

Protective Offense
How Self-Defense Fails Women
and How We Can Fix It

by
Tèja VanWicklen

YMAA Publication Center
Wolfeboro, NH USA

YMAA Publication Center, Inc.
PO Box 480
Wolfeboro, NH 03894
800 669-8892 • www.ymaa.com • info@ymaa.com

ISBN: 9781594399961 (print)
ISBN: 9781594399978 (ebook)
ISBN: 9781594399985 (hardcover)

This book set in Open Sans and Adobe Garamond.

Copyright © 2026 by Tèja VanWicklen
All rights reserved including the right of reproduction in whole or in part in any form. Any use of this intellectual property for text and data mining or computational analysis including as training material for artificial intelligence systems is strictly prohibited without express written consent. For permission requests, contact the Publisher.

Edited by Doran Hunter
Cover design by Axie Breen
Cover illustration by Rina Hyseni, cover concept by Teja VanWicklen
Self-defense illustrations by Joey Docil
Charts by Tahis Fonseca-Miranda

20260206

Publisher's Cataloging in Publication

Names: VanWicklen, Tèja, author. | Miller, Rory Kane, writer of foreword.
Title: Reimagining women's self-defense : protective offense: how self-defense fails women and how we can fix it / Tèja VanWicklen.
Description: Wolfeboro, NH USA : YMAA Publication Center, [2026] | Includes bibliographical references and index.
Identifiers: LCCN: 2025945500 | ISBN: 9781594399985 (hardcover) | 9781594399961 (paperback) | 9781594399978 (ebook)
Subjects: LCSH: Self-defense for women--Handbooks, manuals, etc. | Situational awareness--Safety measures. | Safety education--Handbooks, manuals, etc. | Self-protective behavior--Handbooks, manuals, etc. | Hand-to-hand fighting--Handbooks, manuals, etc. | Crime prevention--Psychological aspects--Handbooks, manuals, etc. | Martial arts--Handbooks, manuals, etc. | BISAC: SELF-HELP / Safety & Security / Personal Safety & Self-Defense. | HEALTH & FITNESS / Women's Health. | SOCIAL SCIENCE / Violence in Society. | SOCIAL SCIENCE / Sexual Abuse & Harassment. | SPORTS & RECREATION / Martial Arts / General.
Classification: LCC: GV1111.5 .V36 2026 | DDC: 613.6/6082--dc23

The author and publisher of the material are NOT RESPONSIBLE in any manner whatsoever for any injury which may occur through reading or following the instructions in this manual.

The activities physical or otherwise, described in this manual may be too strenuous or dangerous for some people, and the reader(s) should consult a physician before engaging in them.

Neither the authors nor the publisher assumes any responsibility for the use or misuse of information contained in this book.

Nothing in this document constitutes a legal opinion nor should any of its contents be treated as such. While the authors believe that everything herein is accurate, any questions regarding specific self-defense situations, legal liability, and/or interpretation of federal, state, or local laws should always be addressed by an attorney at law.

When it comes to martial arts, self-defense, and related topics, no text, no matter how well written, can substitute for professional, hands-on instruction. These materials should be used for academic study only.

Printed in USA.

This book is full of words, yet now they escape me.
Kevin, Zane, you are everything.
And also… to all the women who deserve better.

Contents

Foreword by Rory Miller   xi
Introduction   xiii
    Why This Book?   xiii
    Who Is This Book For?   xvi
    What to Expect   xvii
    How to Use This Book   xx
    Before We Begin   xx

Part 1: PARADIGM SHIFT
Chapter 1: Protective Offense   3
    Shortcomings of Martial-Arts-Based Women's Self-Defense   4
    Protective Offense: The New Self-Defense   8
    Suggested Practices   9

Part 2: SET YOUR MIND
Chapter 2: Me, Myself, and Conflict   15
    The Observer Effect   17
    Zen and the Art of Conflict   19
    The Three-Headed Monster   23
    Flip the Script   25
    Mind-Setting Part 1   30
    Awareness Part 1: Pay Attention!   31
    Recap   33
    Suggested Practices   35

Chapter 3: Where Wolf?   37
    Acceptance and Pragmatism   38
    Common Ground   40
    Scary People   42
    Concepts and Models   45

Social vs. Asocial Violence	50
Recap	52
Suggested Practice	53

Chapter 4: Prey or Privilege — 55
Mind-Setting Part 2	55
Twelve Traits of Protective Offense	57
Recap	62
Suggested Practices	62

Part 3: THE SELF-DEFENSE CONTINUUM

Chapter 5: The Self-Defense Continuum—Overview — 69
Recap	75
Suggested Practices	76

Chapter 6: The Self-Defense Continuum, Stage 1—Decide to Recognize Intent — 77
Awareness Part 2: You See But You Do Not Observe	79
Nonverbal Deception	82
Verbal Deception	92
Devious Tactics	93
Wanting	96
The Safe Category	97
Setting Boundaries	97
Recap	101
Suggested Practice	103

Chapter 7: The Self-Defense Continuum, Stage 2—Deter the Interview — 105
On the Fringe	107
Marc MacYoung's Five Interview Strategies	109
More Devious Tactics	111
Deter by De-escalation	114
Peyton Quinn's Rules of Escalation-Avoidance	116
Recap	119
Suggested Practices	120

Chapter 8: The Self-Defense Continuum, Stage 3—Disrupt Positioning — 123
- Marc MacYoung's Five Positioning Strategies — 124
- Nonviolent Disruption at the Positioning Stage — 127
  - Make Like a Tree — 128
  - Do Voices Carry? — 129
- Recap — 130
- Suggested Practices — 131

Chapter 9: The Self-Defense Continuum, Stage 4—Disengage the Attack — 133
- The Unfair Fight — 134
- The Grand Dilemma — 135
- Deep Self-Trust — 135
- Willing and Able — 137
- Self-Defense Law 101 — 141
- The Three Fs (and Then Some) — 144
- Fight Theory — 147
  - Seven Rules of Disengagement — 148
  - Weapons — 156
  - Basic Protective Techniques and Concepts — 162
  - Other Commonly Taught Self-Defense Techniques — 170
  - Concepts — 178
  - Train Intelligently—Seven Training Tips of Protective Offense — 190
- Recap — 194
- Suggested Practices — 199

Chapter 10: The Self-Defense Continuum, Stage 5—Debrief After the Reaction — 203
- Mental Models and a PTSD-Resistant Mindset — 205
- The Early Debrief — 206
  - Phase 1: Gather Information — 206
  - Phase 2: Assess for Injury — 209
  - Phase 3: Preserve and Collect Evidence — 210
  - Phase 4: Seek Services — 211
- Mid- to Long-Term Debrief — 212
  - A Safe Space — 215
  - Intelligent Healing — 217

Recap	230
Suggested Practices	231

Part 4: THEORY AND PRACTICE

Chapter 11: Continuing Education — 237

Martial Arts, Self-Defense, and Other Alternatives to Investigate in Your Search for Protective Offense	241
Reading Nook	250
Playtime	251
Parent Playtime	256
Play Doctor	257
A Final Word on Continuing Your Education	266

Chapter 12: Reimagining Women's Self-Defense — 267

The Ten Principles of Protective Offense	267

Acknowledgements	273
Bibliography	275
Index	281
About the Author	287

Foreword by Rory Miller

Tèja VanWicklen has been a big influence on me and my work.

The first time we met, I was a rookie on the seminar circuit, and Tèja joined a training in Boston. She'd been a competitive martial artist, managed an international demo team, and studied under tough instructors in rough schools. Eight months into a difficult pregnancy she realized she couldn't perform any of her high-end skills. No one had ever prepared her to work from this level of disadvantage. When she was most vulnerable, most likely to be targeted, all her training was virtually useless.

Another martial artist, another person, would have thrown her hands up or turned exclusively to the gun—not Tèja. She told me she had to rethink everything from the ground up. That was the journey she was on when we met.

If you are a sports martial artist, there is almost nothing you can learn fighting in your own weight class that will be useful to a female self-defense student. Imagine someone twice your size, three times your strength, and with more experience with violence than you. Then imagine this nightmare opponent gets the first move at the time and place of his choosing. This was where Tèja lived and thought from, where she worked problems from—every day.

One of the most profound times Tèja adjusted my thinking was when a few of us were talking about how bad guys get and keep control of their victims—how they psych victims into not fighting back. She said that in real time, there's this moment when a woman has this sudden, shocking realization that things are about to go bad—really, really bad. That she will actually have to fight for her life. She hits him, but not hard—she's terrified of making things worse. He hits her back—and it's devastating—she may never have been hit before—she's frozen, bracing for the beating of her life. Instead, there's this gentle hand, "I'm sorry, honey, I didn't want to do that. Just do what I say, and I promise

I won't hurt you." She knows it's a lie, but in the space between fear and hope, she goes along with it. And then it's too late.

For years, Tèja has been a valuable reality check for me. She has spent the last few decades creating a framework and teaching tools so instructors can reimagine women's self-defense, and so more women can learn to answer their own questions. If you teach self-defense, especially from the point of view of a fit martial athlete, you need her perspective.

>Rory Miller, Author of *Meditations on Violence, Facing Violence,* and *Conflict Communication*
>SW Washington State
>March 2025

Introduction

Why This Book?

I grew up in New York City's East Village before it was trendy. Drug dealers did their business from my stoop while Hell's Angels straddled their Harleys at the curb. The neighborhood was in constant motion. My mother was my only caregiver. She was often sick, and I had no family nearby. When my mother was well, she threw house parties often involving recreational drugs and naked people in our kitchen bathtub (a quirk of old New York City tenements). I experienced sexual abuse at five years old and bullying in school that forced me to leave junior high two weeks before graduation for my safety.

At fifteen, I discovered taekwondo the way some find true love—fireworks and all. Every day after high school I walked two blocks to S. Henry Cho's, climbed the stairs, and sat, cross-legged, in the dusty wooden two-tiered bleachers that overlooked the practice floor. There, I did my homework while Master Cho shuffled papers in the office until the first class began. After sweating through hundreds of crunches, punches, and kicks, I would leave reluctantly at 9 pm. If allowed, I would have slept there.

I learned to do magic on that old chewed-up ocher carpet, to spin and fly and hit the heavy bag harder than anyone thought a 105-pound girl could. I won tournaments. Then grand championships. Coming home at midnight from competitions in neighboring New Jersey, or even as far as Washington, DC, wasn't a problem, I had been navigating the city on my own since I was six. But as I got older, smiles and winks turned to heckling or worse, whispers I could hardly make sense of that set my blood on ice.

As I moved up in the ranks, I repetitively practiced pretty techniques I came to realize would never work for me if one of the whisperers ever got physical. More than once, a tipsy acquaintance at a party grabbed me or held me down, teasing "go ahead, kick my ass," as if it were a pick-up line. Once one of them backed me up threateningly, telling me it was time we got serious and describing how things were going to go this time. When talking didn't work, I spun and kicked him in the gut with the kick I broke six unspaced pine boards with. He exhaled hard, "Nice kick." That was the moment I began questioning every detail of my training.

When I was around twenty, a man who had lived upstairs from me for all but the first two years of my life, and with whom I shared a birthday, was murdered in my building, chopped into pieces, and discarded in garbage bags under my steps. Any remaining semblance of youthful innocence was abruptly and brutally cut off. My mind worked furiously, trying to figure out if and how martial arts could have helped my friend stay alive.

Years later, I would find myself in the backwoods of Pennsylvania studying Sayoc Kali, a Filipino tribal art specializing in edged weapons, martial science, and survival skills. We spent long weekends training with every imaginable weapon on little to no food or sleep, challenging the limits of our physical and mental fortitude. Occasionally, a group of elite military personnel would join us because Pamana Tuhon Christopher C. Sayoc Sr.[1] and the instructors under him were world-class edged weapons experts. I became an emergency medical technician to bolster my training and to be available to others when we were out of range of emergency services. I was loving every second and had begun the process of becoming certified to train military and law enforcement personnel when I became pregnant.

Being pregnant was like stepping into another dimension; there were all these other pregnant women around me who I hadn't noticed before, and kids everywhere, jabbering away, distracting everyone around them, completely helpless but for the guiding hands of their exhausted parents. On top of the mental shift, my body became entirely foreign to me. I was so nauseated and rundown in my first two trimesters that I

---

[1] "Pamana" means "heritage" or "legacy" in Tagalog, but within the Sayoc tribe it carries deeper weight. Pamana Tuhon Christopher C. Sayoc Sr. established the title "Tuhon" as a rank rooted in blood, sacrifice, and earned mastery. Others have appropriated the term without understanding its history; the true Tuhon rank begins and ends with the Sayoc legacy and is considered a sacred inheritance.

couldn't work out. I developed an inguinal hernia in my third trimester that required surgery and bedrest; labor went on for several grueling days, leaving me physically incapable of sleep and shaking like a trapped animal. The gauntlet continued with other anomalous issues and conditions. I mourned the loss of my previously dependable physical health as I watched hard-earned muscle dissolve and I became weak and uncoordinated.

Physically diminished and distracted by my unremitting responsibility to this tiny, fragile, new being, it seemed that my martial arts training no longer applied. I searched my databanks: when had training ever covered fleeing from danger with a stroller in tow or fighting off a determined mugger while wearing a baby in a carrier as body armor? What were the answers to any number of extremely disturbing scenarios? I had dedicated my life to the art and instruction of self-defense and somehow missed crucial, everyday reference points. Didn't lots of people have children? Injuries? Extenuating circumstances?

I was consistently asked where to go for self-defense training or what martial art to study and had no satisfactory answers. It seemed odd that there was a need but no consistent message or even a generally agreed-upon framework. I ran through the encyclopedia of fighting techniques in my head—scrutinized them in multiple scenarios, talked to everyone, and cross-referenced between martial systems. The more I focused on fight techniques, the clearer it became that physical self-defense was at the end of a continuum and that other skill sets needed to take precedence. A self-defense timeline began to evolve and with it a recognition of the need for pragmatic skills to empower women to take ownership of their own and their family's safety.

It was at about this time that, in my quest to find others who were examining the less-obvious aspects of violence, conflict, and self-defense, I met Erik Kondo who recommended I read Rory Miller's book *Meditations on Violence*. Soon after, Erik ran one of Rory's early seminars. Rory and I began a correspondence, then a friendship. Rory, Marc MacYoung, Erik Kondo, Kathy Jackson, Garry Smith, Clint Overland, Toby Cowern, Terry Trahan, and I formed a kind of thinktank we dubbed Conflict Research Group International (CRGI), which became an online magazine. Over several years we cracked open quandaries that remained even after decades in the martial arts—unsolved mysteries, pet peeves, random curiosities, deep questions—all in the name of deciphering conflict, violence, and predatory behaviors. We chewed the meat off the bone and then we chewed the bone some more.

This book began as notes to myself and grew into a kind of framework for all the skill sets I was trying to fit into my life as a mother, student, and instructor. I wrote to map the inaccurately charted territory of women's self-defense training; I wrote to dissect what I felt were innate problems with the applicability of many techniques and to find a deeper, more informed empowerment than the kind that came with blindly believing I could kick ass. I used the initial work to create the Secrets of Women's Self-Defense course that ran online at Women's Wellness University, a community of over a hundred thousand women.

> … *find everything interesting… curiosity, awareness, attention. Those are the tools we need if we hope to avoid the worst mistakes, and, indeed, if our children are to have a future on this planet.*
> —Laurence Gonzales, from his book *Everyday Survival*

Who Is This Book For?

This book is primarily for martial arts and self-defense instructors, seasoned practitioners, safety and security professionals, and conflict analysts interested in emptying their cups and starting from scratch without all the institutional, political, and tribal baggage gathered from the martial arts world; it's for those asking more intentional questions: which mental and physical skills do we most need so we can protect ourselves and our kids when we're alone with them? What can we do if we're ill, injured, pregnant, or otherwise impaired? What if our kids or students want to party intelligently or are simply curious about how predators think and what they look for in a victim?

Despite the many self-defense books for women, it feels like we are screaming into a void. Not enough women are reading, not enough are gaining protective skill sets and passing them on. Perhaps it's because most of the women's self-defense books are written by men who, though well-intentioned, fail to grasp the deepest, darkest, most gut-wrenching aspects of being female. It's up to instructors to put ego aside, figure out what is missing, and collaborate and learn rather than just continue to teach what we have always taught.

Women are not the only vulnerable population; those in the LGBTQIA+ community are at similar risk; depending on the statistics you look at, the risk to young boys may only be slightly lower. Erik Kondo is a paraplegic jiu-jitsu instructor who understands the vulnerabilities of those in the disabled world and we have often discussed similarities between women's self-defense and self-defense for other vulnerable groups.

Perhaps we can reimagine self-defense if we put tradition and tribalism aside for a just a moment, forget which is the coolest technique or concept, and reexamine the subject matter with a focus on how best to serve the populations who need us most.

What to Expect

I believe men practice martial arts for love of the arts, camaraderie, competition, aggression management, and for general fitness or to break up their gym workout. I believe women and people of the queer and nonbinary communities do it for those same reasons and more:

- general empowerment
- anxiety over past or ongoing trauma and troubling events that have happened to them or to someone they know
- real concerns of potential danger
- unnamed anxiety that defies the usual solutions; feeling constantly vulnerable for no apparent reason; hypervigilance
- a friend or family member suggested a self-defense class as an antidote to the above issues

The majority of these involve anxiety, all of them if you think of empowerment at least partly as the mitigation of anxiety. It is important to note that even unnamed anxiety is not always without foundation. Women are generally more at risk in daily life, more aware of danger, and arguably more connected to their mortality than men are. Whether this is due to our biological connection to life, being smaller, physically weaker, and having less social or political power than our male counterparts, or that we are often responsible for others—we just worry about safety more often than the average guy. Ask a man how often he thinks about safety or worries about going out alone, then ask a woman or queer person the same question.

> In the research article, "Gender-Based Heat Map Images of Campus Walking Settings," researchers found that women focused on a wider visual range than men, specifically areas outside the path they were walking on.[2]

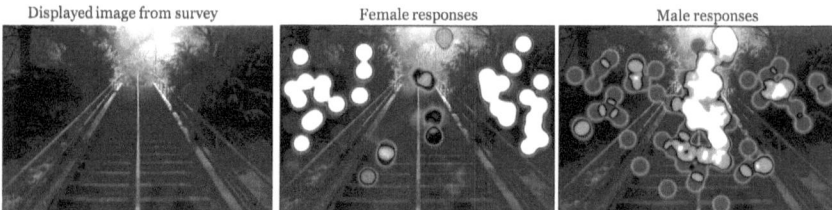

Whether you came to this book to become a more effective self-defense instructor or to feel safer and allay some of the hypervigilance that often comes with being female, I hope you will come away as a more astute, self-aware, resilient, informed, and abuse-resistant version of yourself, and with a new vocabulary for self-defense.

Though this book does cover some specifics of parenthood, it is geared toward a broader range of women. Many, if not all, the skills herein apply to single moms of multiples with strollers and carriers, but I leave the most parent-specific skills for another book. If you are responsible for children or dependents, you will find more than enough to get started.

---

2 Robert A. Chaney, Alyssa Baer, and L. Ida Tovar. 2023. "Gender-Based Heat Map Images of Campus Walking Settings: A Reflection of Lived Experience." *Violence and Gender* 11 (1): 35–42. https://doi.org/10.1089/vio.2023.0027.

Introduction

Learn To:
- break down the process of violent crime
- stay off the criminal radar
- recognize the signs, tells, and tricks of emotionally abusive people and violent criminals
- respond as early as possible to a confrontation by multiple attackers
- consider how weapons can be used and what your options are if confronted by them
- navigate confusion and shock under duress
- know which physical techniques to count on in a fight for your life
- know which physical techniques NOT to count on in a fight for your life
- grasp the most important legal ramifications of physically protecting yourself against violence
- vet a litany of self-defense techniques accounting for size, strength, skills, and lifestyle
- include specific considerations of parenthood in your self-defense practice
- model an aware and proactive mindset for children
- evaluate self-defense techniques and make them your own
- evaluate self-defense courses and instructors and make educated decisions about who to trust with your training and your family's training
- begin thinking about how to raise children who will never present themselves as unsuspecting targets, and who will never victimize others
- connect intimately to your intuition so you can use it in your calculations without concern that you're not being logical
- heal intelligently after a violent encounter
- use the book's tools and resources to become a more effective coach
- engage and encourage others to reimagine women's self-defense training, so it benefits us all

How to Use This Book

Read it linearly the way it was written. Go straight to the chapters that interest you. Browse it as a guide. Check it as a reference. Though the chronology of the chapters is important, it shouldn't deter you from reading the parts that interest you first. Do it your way. Unless your instructor assigned it, in which case, do it her way.

Throughout this book, I will use the words criminal, predator, attacker, assailant, threat, bad guy, and troublemaker. Whenever I use these terms, always assume I mean more than one person.

I use "he," "she," and "they" interchangeably, though I use "he, him" pronouns most often when referring to an imagined criminal to simplify because, statistically, there are far more male criminals than other genders. I use "she, her" pronouns to refer to all those who identify as women.

When I refer to "martial arts" I mean a systematized method of combat training; when I refer to "self-defense," I mean a way for people to protect themselves that may draw on a number of martial arts and other skills, or a legal term indicating the reason you felt it was required for you to hurt someone.

I will explain the term "protective offense" in the next chapter and will use the terms self-defense and protective offense interchangeably throughout the book.

Before We Begin

As a neglected child raised around drugs and violence, a life-long martial artist with a background in edged weapons, firearms, wilderness survival, emergency management, and personal training, and as a mother who endured a grueling pregnancy and over a year of post-partum health issues, I navigate the unpredictable terrain of predators and their unsuspecting targets specifically for women. I have tried many things I don't necessarily recommend you try and had experiences I might have been happier—though not necessarily smarter—without. I have trained with some unusual thinkers, read avidly, questioned everything and everyone and, I hope, ended up with a workable contextual

Introduction

picture of how danger, self-defense, conflict, and personal emergency management work in real time.

This book is filled with wisdom I've collected over many years from violence professionals, conflict analysts, and the study of psychology, survival, PTSD, etc. I thank all those who came before me, all those who sacrificed, and all those who continue to do the complex work of analyzing conflict and violence often at their own risk.

Reimagining Women's Self-Defense is my contribution to the overall project of equality, safety, and dynamic living for women and families. Until many more of us can truly protect ourselves and our loved ones, women will remain second-class citizens. I sincerely hope this book will change the way people view and discuss women's self-defense. That said, there is no one-size-fits-all answer for anyone, and I wish only to begin a discussion. What follows is based on my own experiences, not a treatise on how others should live or train. Fighting is only one tenth of self-defense, but it hoards 90 percent of the spotlight. There is so much more women can do to protect themselves from the rougher side of life than just kick and punch.

Life is a journey. To the well-informed traveler, danger is simply a call to adventure.

PART 1

PARADIGM SHIFT

CHAPTER 1

Protective Offense

*We cannot solve our problems with the same thinking
we used to create them.*
　　　　　—Attributed to both Ram Dass and Albert Einstein

Two thousand years ago, when the martial arts were evolving, women's empowerment and freedom of movement weren't high on the agenda, yet women are still learning ancient self-defense concepts originally designed by and for men.

I've had a love/hate relationship with martial arts for over thirty years. I revel in the training and the adrenaline rush, but I'm frustrated by techniques that don't seem adapted to my body or my circumstances and by the backlash from the establishment that occurs whenever I express thoughts that deviate from the doctrine.

With a modern overhaul of women's self-defense more women might become students and instructors. Parents might share protective knowledge and techniques with children through stories and play the way some indigenous cultures still do. We might see a decrease—if not in attempted violence—perhaps in successful violence against women.

I see classes and seminars where, through role-play, women learn the simple tells and tricks of emotionally unstable people and hardened criminals. Students would learn that anyone who disregards a firm "no" should be cut off from further interaction. Girls would understand the many ploys a criminal might use to distract her or get her to share a ride. A freshman letting loose her first weeks in college would know that no matter how good-looking or charming a man might seem, he could still be a predator, and though he appears to know her friends he may simply be an excellent listener. She would know the statistics are loud and clear that once she is in that car, she's going to a place of the criminal's choosing and might not be coming back. She would also know how to fight using every object in reach as a weapon should anyone ever pull a knife and try to coerce her into a bad situation without her consent.

Could women's self-defense be failing those who need it most? If so, what ails it? A dependence on ancient techniques? A disconnect between teacher and student? Reluctance to go back to the drawing board? Or all the above and more?

> *A lie that is being promoted is that sport-based martial arts training IS self-defense training. This lie has become so endemic it is accepted as "the truth"—that's until you end up bleeding or arrested because you discovered firsthand they aren't the same. When it comes to the realities of staying safe in a modern urban environment… your personal safety will be far better served by understanding crime and home security and avoiding high-risk behaviors than by being able to break a board with your big toe.*
> —Marc MacYoung, conflict analyst, author, expert witness

Shortcomings of Martial-Arts-Based Women's Self-Defense

Let's be clear: martial arts and self-defense are not the same things. Martial arts are combat arts—combat and art being the operative terms. They are predominantly physical methods of fighting, often face-to-face.

Chapter 1: Protective Offense

They are systematized and often practiced by rote. They are fun, they can be very useful, but they are only partly or indirectly translatable to self-defense. Self-defense is not about mastering a number of technical skills, it is about understanding predatory tactics in the name of avoidance, and, if necessary, ending a fight as quickly as possible and being physically able to walk away. However…

- **Many modern self-defense techniques have their origins in ancient combat arts** often involving antiquated weapons and even horseback. These have been handed down mostly unchanged over generations, creating self-defense that often feels retrofitted to suit the needs of modern women though it was originally built for an entirely different purpose.
- **Most martial arts were created by and for men** and are therefore specific to a man's biology and lifestyle. These arts neglect crucial issues like pregnancy and strollers and fail to grasp the devastating implications of vast differences in height, strength, and leverage.
- **Instructors may only have a superficial understanding of their student's experiences of danger and assault.** Some instructors have military or law-enforcement backgrounds which, though appearing to correspond to self-defense needs, involve vastly different rules and goals.
- **Many modern classes focus predominantly on fair fights** where two consenting people—often of about the same size and weight—face off against one another. This does not even vaguely mimic a criminal interaction and can put women at a fatal disadvantage.
- **Instruction is often disconnected from everyday realities** like parenthood, overwork, physical disability, sleep deprivation, age, and illness. For reasons related to insurance premiums and convenience, self-defense is nearly always practiced by people in comfortable clothing on smooth floors in a well-lit environment free of obstacles. Training within contextualized scenarios is rare. Screaming children, shopping bags, heavy, restrictive winter clothing, high-heeled shoes, uneven terrain, darkness, wind, rain, and speeding traffic must be part of an instructor's consciousness or self-defense training will be as useful as learning to drive exclusively by playing a video game.

- **The spectacle of stunt-heavy Hollywood movies and sports martial arts confuse us into adopting finesse techniques that are more elegant or acrobatic than practical.** These techniques often require too much time and physical space when an attacker may be right on top of you. The mind and body respond very differently under extreme stress, and we are unlikely to be able to execute a series of intricate movements under duress, even with years of practice.
- **Training can be unhealthy for our bodies,** causing chronic shoulder, knee, and back injuries that ironically make it more difficult for us to protect ourselves.
- **Training is often over-focused on the moment of attack** and neglects skills like deterrence, intent recognition, and de-escalation, which can diminish our presence on the criminal radar.
- **Those in need of training may be least likely to seek it out.** Classes are often filled with type-A personalities—people who are naturally inclined toward physical fitness and assertiveness. Women often only look for answers after they have been attacked. Those who have been traumatized, don't exercise, or are naturally shy may be intimidated or overwhelmed.
- **Often, people seeking training don't find themselves represented by their instructors.** Legal scholar and author Mary Ann Franks says, "White men have never been the primary targets of violent crime, and yet it is their interests and their view of the world that dominates not only the legal but the social understanding of self-defense."
- **The accepted pseudo-military structure of many martial arts classes may encourage subservience.** This is at odds with the truth that asking questions and formulating ideas are skills indispensable to our general safety. Worse, the systematic discouragement of natural inquisitiveness is detrimental to young women who must learn to trust themselves to be safe. An instructor must be a guide and role model, not a disciplinarian. And a role model should *never* discourage us from exploring and forming ideas about our own protection.

Those are the obvious issues, but there are others. Instructors will talk about self-defense being 90 percent mental, but too often the training doesn't reflect the assertion. That's because teaching students to cultivate self-awareness in a way that enables them to fix glitches is difficult; it doesn't provide an obvious goal or lend itself to progress tracking. It is said that there are more combinations of chess pieces on a board than atoms in the universe. The same is true of the variety of possible crime scenarios. No number of physical techniques alone will answer all the variations.

People engage in martial arts and self-defense to feel empowered, but the concept is misunderstood and the word misused. Blind or reckless empowerment may cause us to become overly assertive. We love to hear about the grandma who fought off the attacker who tried to take her purse, but there are many versions of this story that went badly. We must literally choose our battles or we risk sacrificing ourselves for a bit of spare change. Physical empowerment in the absence of contextual and experiential knowledge can cause us to jump into situations we aren't ready to handle. Lack of understanding about the various stages of an emergency can mean we wade in too deeply before realizing we had other options. Empowerment must be informed.

Women are not only generally smaller and weaker than their attackers; we are conditioned to react to threats and coercion with social behavior, like kindness or self-deprecation. A woman might be pregnant or responsible for multiple children. Gangs or college fraternities might team up against unsuspecting, weaker individuals.

For these reasons and more, women's self-defense is long overdue for an evolutionary jump. In architecture, buildings are designed around the people who live or work there; we don't build hospitals the same way we build homes or libraries. Currently, women's self-defense is a version of men's self-defense, but it should be a different species altogether; both can have two eyes and a nose, but for women to protect themselves against larger, stronger, more experienced opponents with better leverage, weapons, and the element of surprise, we don't just need a taller ladder—we need wings.

Protective Offense: The New Self-Defense

The best defense is a good offense.
—Attributed to George Washington

If we are reinventing women's self-defense to include others we care for beyond just ourselves—if we are creating a more proactive and empowering mindset—couldn't we find a term that better reflects these updates?

For a long time, I have taken issue with the term self-defense. "Self" leaves out others we are responsible for and "defense" sounds too passive or reactionary. "Self-defense" is the legal term that describes to a judge why you hit your assailant with a baseball bat. It does not describe a group of skills we need to protect ourselves from violence. We need a term that is both empowering and inclusive of family members who need us.

I've been using the term "protective offense" for nearly twenty years. Protective offense is offense for the purpose of self-defense, offense as in chess or sports—thinking several steps ahead, being aware of patterns, and out-strategizing your opponent. To go on the offense is to take control of circumstances. A good defense can be part of an offensive strategy, like building a wall around a castle. But how long can you defend against a hoard of attackers, or even one wielding a knife, before you are too tired or injured to continue? The word "defense" works in legal terminology but not as a mindset or goal during a life-threatening attack.

Expanding to meet the needs of women, families, and other vulnerable populations means protective offense must go way beyond the study of fighting; it must consider the big picture—the before, during, and after of crime—as well as general emergency management. Vulnerability is the number-one quality predators look for. It is our job to be aware of our vulnerabilities and to minimize or find strength in them.

Strength is my weakness? How can strength be my weakness!
—Kevin Hart in *Jumanji: Welcome to the Jungle*

Fighting means risking damage. Even successfully warding off a rapist can leave you emotionally scarred for years. If you have a child or dependent with you, avoiding a physical altercation is even more urgent. Learning to physically fight is one tool in your bag, but it shouldn't be the only one. How do we allow an unstable person to back out of an altercation without embarrassment? Can we read the body language of someone who is quietly telling us they intend harm? Who at the office is genuine and who has ulterior motives? How do we undertake prevention, deterrence, and de-escalation? Subtle levels of communication play a large role in conflict and in life. The same training that teaches us to avoid predators can teach us to avoid all manners of unpleasant interactions.

Protective offense is the study of people-reading and conflict management, of self- and situational awareness, de-escalation, and high-speed problem solving—it's a road to dynamic rather than passive or fearful living. Protective offense helps us see in greater detail, make more effective decisions, and go out into the world better prepared for all of life's sudden curves.

Suggested Practices

These exercises are designed to help you wring all the juice out of this book. Here are some ways you can begin to explore protective offense.

 Non-judgmental journaling. You've probably been encouraged to keep a journal by everyone from your parents to your psychologist. That's because journaling accomplishes many things at once: it helps us bring miscellaneous worries to the front of the brain where we can address and release them; it's a place to track dreams, which sometimes tell us what we are really thinking about; it's a great way to keep an eye on emotional trends by identifying patterns of ingrained behavior—something we pay therapists a lot of money to do. Journaling may not be a substitute for a psychologist, but it may afford us some of the benefits without one. If you have a psychologist, journaling can make your doctor's job and yours easier and more efficient. A journal allows you to look back and see which exercises or modalities made you more effective. And there's no better motivational tool than seeing improvement.

A paragraph or so may be all you need—even a few sentences will do. Flowing ideas are probably best, but you can use bullet points or short hand if that works better for you. Make it as easy as possible: put a notebook and pen by your bed, or use your phone or tablet to type or dictate. Just write, don't judge.

Keeping a journal may serve you during the reading of this book. And if you ever decide to write your memoirs, you'll have it handy to trigger important memories that might have otherwise been lost.

 Navigate your home blindfolded. In the event of a nighttime emergency like a fire or a blackout, you will want to find your way to your children or to the doors without panicking. Fear galvanizes; panic paralyzes. Knowing how to deal with darkness can go a long way toward helping you find and maintain calm under pressure.

Sighted people lean heavily on this one sense. Spending a longer than comfortable period without your sight to guide you forces you to rely on your other senses. You may feel unbalanced and disoriented. The urge to peek might be very strong. For safety, go slowly and have a friend or family member close by.

There are indigenous forest tracking methods that teach you to walk in the dark silently and accident-free. We can take some pointers from them as well as from the internal martial arts. Don't lean too far forward or back, and stay centered and balanced over your feet. Keep your knees soft, and don't lock them or tense your body, which will only throw off your balance. Take your time and try to hear and feel your environment. Don't rush. Think of this exercise as a kind of moving meditation.

You have a choice of techniques. You can pick your feet up a few inches off the floor as though you are stepping over something. This will help give notice if something is in your way; it will slow you down and, as an added benefit, remind you to concentrate on balance. If you have an injury or trouble with balance, try sliding one foot forward at a time. Keep contact with the floor and when you find an obstacle, work around it. Never heel-toe but reach out more with the ball of the foot, which becomes much more important without your eyes. Make sure you know what's in front of you before you commit your full weight. If you're going up or down stairs, be especially slow and cautious.

This practice exercises balance, patience, hearing, intuition, focus, kinesthetic awareness, and a slew of small muscles that rarely get enough attention. It will make you more intimate with the place where you spend a large proportion of your life.

PART 2
SET YOUR MIND

CHAPTER 2

Me, Myself, and Conflict

Wherever you go, there you are.
  —Often attributed to Buckaroo Bansai

It was another critical election, and I didn't want to just sit on my ass, so I drove upstate to volunteer for *Get Out the Vote* figuring I would kill two birds with one stone and visit friends afterward. When I arrived, ready for my first polling experience, there was no one to partner with and they asked if I minded going out alone. This was unusual. There were strict safety protocols around partnering and nighttime polling—or so I was told on the phone. When I arrived, however, everyone was on fire to make a last-minute difference. Eager to help, I jumped back in the car with a list of registered voters and my GPS as the sky began to darken.

I'm a born and raised city girl who nonetheless loves fresh air and open spaces, but the country is not my natural habitat. As I followed winding roads out of town, houses spread to fifty feet apart and sat twenty to forty feet off treelined streets. By now it was nearly pitch dark with only the occasional garage motion sensor throwing a circle of light at the ground. Checking my list to ensure the numbers matched, I parked, stepped out of the car, and headed up the driveway. Halfway to the house, I froze. In the deep shadows beneath the evergreens and at the base of a deck about forty feet in front of me sat what appeared to be a statue of a stocky, medium-sized dog.

It was at that moment that I recognized my error. I had forgone my standard operating procedure—I was in unfamiliar territory behaving as if it were familiar. I should have pulled into the long driveway rather than left the car down at the street. As I turned to sidle toward the car, the dark statue rose onto all fours and began moving silently toward me. As in a horror film, shadows seemed to thicken. My mind emptied. I knew any sudden motion would trigger the chase instinct. I took long, slow steps, trying to outpace the danger without moving quickly. Instinct or training had finally kicked in. I heard myself yell sharply—not the cry of a scared or wounded animal but the staccato "HEY!" of a trainer redirecting behavior. The shadow stopped abruptly if only for a moment. I tried my trick again and the creature paused. I made it to my car with about twelve feet to spare.

Safe inside, I turned and saw the dark figure hovering just beyond the red taillight of my SUV. It retreated before I could get a good look at it. And I was already trying to forget.

It's beyond irksome that errors like this persist despite so many years of training. I could go on and talk about other lapses, like the time I locked my infant son in the car while it was running. We're not supposed to do this as professionals. We're supposed to appear bulletproof—to show others what they can become with a little knowledge and focus. But I believe honesty is more important.

The study of protective offense is an ongoing process. We will make mistakes. We will even make the same mistakes again. Hopefully, because our training buffered us, those mistakes will become lessons and won't be the worst—or last—mistakes of our lives.

Everything we do as instructors (and parents) matters. We work on ourselves, model behavior for our students (and children), and everything flows from there. We can only assume that the better we understand our own mental glitches and the mechanics of the mishap, the more practice we have managing adrenaline and thinking under stress, the clearer and more impactful our teaching and the higher our level of personal safety and quality of life.

The dog should have been tied up or locked in the house, the volunteer organization should have stuck to its safety protocols—we can always point to others, there is more than enough blame to go around. But it was my ass on the line, my son waiting for me at home, and I let overconfidence and a blind need to feel good about being of service put me in the danger zone.

> *Trouble doesn't happen to us, it happens because of us.*
> —Karim Hajee, life coach, author

The Observer Effect

We are the one constant in any conflict or emergency we face. Just by being there, we alter the course of events—we change the dynamics. This is known as the observer effect: observation changes the thing being observed. Interaction naturally changes it even more, which means our reactions, responses, and decisions matter. The problem is that our thought processes and behaviors are mostly invisible to us.

Much of what we do is by choice. Major life choices are relatively easy to track, but we make hundreds of tiny yet relevant decisions every day: to pack a phone charger, to plan carefully for a long trip or wing it, to stop for gas or wait until we're almost empty. We put the recurring signals of intuition together or we don't. Our lives extend from the micro-choices we either make or don't make. Seemingly inconsequential decisions can impact our position in the world in general and place us on the criminal radar in particular. We should begin our quest for the somewhat opposing goals of personal safety and dynamic living by accepting that our choices matter.

We are by no means singularly responsible for everything that happens to us, but we always play some part. How large a role we play in a crisis can be difficult or even impossible to measure, but our role is relevant and rarely discussed, mainly because it's neither comfortable nor socially acceptable to do so. It is therefore possible for us to be a significant blind spot even as we plan for our personal safety and quality of life. As photographers, we aren't in the pictures, but we are there, affecting the resulting photo through choices of framing, angle, and focus.

If you are a self-defense instructor, your students might say, "Wait a minute, if someone attacks me, I'm not the problem, the bad guy is. End of discussion." They're right, of course, but being right won't keep crises from happening or help you teach them anything of substance. We are not placing blame; blame is a useless concept that only blurs everyone's ability to focus on the big picture. We must drain emotion from the equation long enough to see the entire issue even if it feels counterintuitive or unfair. These are emotionally charged issues, but solving problems is dirty work, and we need to roll up our sleeves and dig through all the muck, not just some of it. And our own muck is always the most unpleasant to dig through.

Small things often add up before big things go wrong: she was always attracted to creeps, he was always trusting to a fault. We're so used to multi-tasking that we don't look up when we cross the street; we text while driving, we open doors after a knock without looking through the peephole first. We may or may not have control over whether someone steals our identity. It's reasonable to own a credit card, and we must set the bar at a reasonable height. We can check our credit history, shred paper mail, and jump through other hoops, but there are crimes that can be difficult to avoid. Common sense tells us fewer crummy things happen to those who are self-aware and take responsibility for their choices and actions—who learn from previous mistakes, make thoughtful decisions, and listen to those who warn them about recurring lapses in judgment. When we look back on our mistakes honestly, we raise ourselves up to higher ground where we are less likely to look down and find the water at our knees. When we listen to our intuition, use emotions and logic synergistically, and make informed choices, we are likely to escape unfortunate situations sooner and with less bloodshed.

Chapter 2: Me, Myself, and Conflict

...he who hath so little knowledge of human nature as to seek happiness by changing anything but his own disposition, will waste his life in fruitless efforts and multiply the grief he proposes to remove.
—Samuel Johnson, 18th century poet, playwright, moralist

In his seminal work, *The 7 Habits of Highly Effective People*, Steven Covey reminds us of what Epictetus wrote thousands of years before about the Circle of Concern and the Circle of Influence. The Circle of Concern describes everything we dwell on, fuss over, and worry about: other people's attitudes, weather, traffic, our general health and financial situation. The Circle of Influence describes the things we actually have influence over: our own health and financial situation. The simple yet eye-opening point is that we often spend valuable time and energy worrying about things we have no control over rather than focusing on where we can make positive changes.

YOU are the part of the equation you have the most control over. YOU are within your Circle of Influence. To worry about predators and ignore your own contribution to your life story is to drive half a car. Physical protection is only a small part of a much larger picture. It is not the physical technique that makes us safer, it is who we are and how we manage conflict. The greatest teachers impart these principles to their students and children by being their own best students first and modeling behaviors, not by lectures and discipline.

Knowing that we are responsible— "response-able"— is fundamental to effectiveness...
—Stephen Covey, author of *The 7 Habits of Highly Effective People*

Zen and the Art of Conflict

We dream of a life without conflict, but conflict is essential. Like oxygen, it is ever-present, simultaneously building us up and breaking us down. Just the idea of conflict can cause our shoulders to tense, yet without it we lack the challenges that enliven us, lose connection to ourselves and others, and at least figuratively waste away. So much conflict is interwoven throughout life that if we could harness the energy, we might single-handedly light up a small city or launch something into space. Conflict is a slippery, elusive creature, but by understanding our personal relationship to it, we might tame it just a bit.

Conflict comes in many forms. You may be brilliant at pacifying an angry boss but incapable of doing the same with a frustrated toddler. We tend to see all conflict as negative yet it forces us to reach beyond our comfort zone into new challenges. Every day, somewhere, someone turns a negative experience into enlightenment—a non-profit, a book, or even a movement. This requires resilience, the ability to overcome the initial event and ride out the subsequent turbulence. Resilience is one of many tools of conflict management along with self-awareness, reframing, empathy, creativity, patience, integrity, and the ability to spot behavioral patterns, among others.

For me, as a mother and family member, conflict management means navigating the minefield of differing needs, wants, and opinions on a relentless and ongoing basis. As a self-defense analyst, conflict management is the crux. To teach someone to protect themselves and their families without learning to manage conflict is to teach them to pull a trigger without learning basic firearms safety.

How we deal with conflict when it raises its ugly mug is a crucial quality-of-life and even a life-or-death issue. Conflict can turn to full-on emergency if we let it, and emergencies, like black holes, swallow time and options. Even well-handled conflict can leave a scummy residue.

Once we accept that there is no way to eliminate conflict, adversity, and stress from life, we can aspire to become conflict managers, people who are able to mitigate emergencies and even turn conflict to advantage and opportunity.

Conflict creates stress (or vice versa), and stress can have a detrimental effect on our ability to make effective decisions. But not all stress is bad. According to Buddhist thought stress is not internal; it's the mind's negative response to external factors, so the way we think about stress may be worse than the stress itself. In her enlightening TED talk, "How to Make Stress Your Friend," psychologist Kelly McGonigal makes the important point that many types of stress we consider detrimental may only be so because of the way we think about them. She cites a study in which people who thought of their stress as a helpful adaptation—like lifting weights for their nervous system—had no negative results or increase in likelihood of cardiovascular disease associated with stress.[3] Not all stress is bad stress, and even bad stress doesn't always have to be bad *for you*. Popular authors in the health and wellness fields like Ori Hofmekler, author of *The 7 Principles of Stress*, cite the beneficial aspects of stress, like a stronger immune system, which may come from our innate ability to adapt and the subsequent need to work our "adaptation muscles."

Still, stress sometimes overwhelms us, and there are skills we can practice to help us cope in the moment. Self-observation is the first step to self-management. Log your reflexive responses to stressful situations: do you pause, lash out, or freeze when you are stressed or challenged? The ability to self-observe is a miraculous human skill and a primary one in both protective offense and life. Our responses to stress have huge implications, and our children will watch us and mimic our behavior.

> *More is caught than taught.*
> —John Maxwell, American author, leadership speaker, and pastor

Armed with knowledge of how we respond to the world, we can begin to recognize the earliest signs of stress and reframe our circumstances in ways that lead to better outcomes. Framing refers to the picture we create out of the information we have. We can rearrange our frame to include elements that help us make better judgement calls while also confirming that our viewpoint is valid and not based on a false premise. By changing our frame of reference, we can change our emotional responses and the parts of our creative and analytical brains that are accessed.

We might find we are able to reframe certain kinds of stress as excitement. Many symptoms of stress or anxiety (perspiring, racing heart,

---

[3] Abigail Keller et al., "Does the Perception That Stress Affects Health Matter? The Association with Health and Mortality," *Health Psychology* 31, no. 5 (September 2012): 677–84, https://doi.org/10.1037/a0026743.

shaking hands, dry mouth) are virtually identical to the symptoms of excitement. Alison Wood Brooks, assistant professor at Harvard Business School, found that people who reframed pre-performance work anxiety as excitement performed better under stress and that reappraising and reframing negative emotions could be more effective than suppressing them or trying to relax, which often worsened anxiety.[4]

Another way to reframe is to consider the viewpoint of others involved in the conflict. Steven Covey refers to reframing as paradigm shifts in *The 7 Habits of Highly Effective People*. He describes being on a subway surrounded by a band of loud, unruly kids, their father sitting quietly by, allowing the chaos to disrupt other people's lives. Covey finally says something to the father and discovers the man's wife—the children's mother—has just passed away after an extended illness. The kids and the father are all exorcizing their shock in different ways. This realization causes Covey to move from annoyance to empathy.

We can also reframe by imagining someone we respect or care for in our place. By temporarily adopting another persona we can shift our point of reference and devise solutions we hadn't thought of.

Though anxiety can overwhelm our faculties it may also imbue us with productive energy so long as we learn to listen and manage our responses. Armed with knowledge of how we respond to conflict, we can begin to recognize the earliest signs of stress, reframe our circumstances in ways that lead to better outcomes, and even reappraise negative emotions in general as potentially productive rather than detrimental.

> *…for stress defines us and develops us. We are the present product of the past stresses we have experienced…*
> —P. A. Hancock and J. L. Szalma, from *Performance Under Stress: Research Insights for Better Operational Decisions*

---

[4] Alison Wood Brooks, "Get Excited: Reappraising Pre-Performance Anxiety as Excitement," *Journal of Experimental Psychology: General* 143, no. 3 (June 2014): 1144–58, https://doi.org/10.1037/a0035325.

Chapter 2: Me, Myself, and Conflict

The Three-Headed Monster[5]

The Triune Brain Theory, as proposed by neuroscientist Paul D. MacLean in the 1960s, is now seen as an oversimplification and even outright false by many modern scientists, yet it persists because of its applicability as a model. Models are simplified ways of representing complex ideas to enable us to visualize and organize thoughts. The Triune Brain Theory illustrates how different parts of the brain evolved as we faced new issues that arose from proto-human life and lead us to a useful understanding of certain brain functions and behaviors.

In the Triune Brain model, the basal ganglia or lizard brain (though all vertebrates likely possessed it) is the oldest, most survival-centric part of the brain. It evolved to deal with urgent issues of food acquisition, predators, and procreation—what I've heard referred to as the three Fs: Food, Fight, Fuck—the primary business of the times. As we created communities with complex social hierarchies, the paleomammalian complex or limbic system—the monkey brain—evolved. The newest parts of the brain to evolve are referred to collectively as the neo-mammalian complex or neocortex. This is the analytical and abstract thinking brain that builds skyscrapers and invents language and flying machines. This is the part of the brain we think of as most human.

> The Triune Brain theory supplies a simple analogy for brain and nervous system functions that might otherwise be unwieldy or elusive to describe. Analogical thinking, that is, using analogy in cognitive processes, can be a highly useful method for understanding, problem-solving, and teaching. Douglas Richard Hofstadter, Pulitzer prize-winning author and cognitive and computer scientist, said, "Analogy is the core of cognition."[6]

The lizard brain has the power to hijack your entire system—to send you into a burning building to save your child. It is most obvious in moments of extreme fear or stress and is responsible for the cascade of adrenaline and cortisol we call the fight-or-flight response. It is also the

---

5 Rory Miller uses the triune brain theory to deftly explicate human behavior in *Conflict Communication*, the book that incited me to include this important section.
6 Mary L. Gick and Keith J. Holyoak, "Analogical Problem-Solving," *Cognitive Psychology* 12, no. 3 (July 1980): 306–55.

fastest decision-maker by far. The lizard brain goes right to work while the slow human brain plods along trying to figure out what to do next.

When my son was four years old, he hurled himself from the top of a jungle gym while my head was momentarily turned. I still don't know how I caught him in midair—whether I saw motion in my periphery, heard his breath, or saw concern in someone else's eyes. But I surely hadn't done any cognitive calculations.

Abuse or hardship, especially early in life, imprints on the lizard brain and hardwires emotional and physical responses, making them extremely resistant to change.

The monkey brain is the social-emotional center—the part of the brain that gets us into the most trouble. When it evolved, social status dictated how resources were allocated and whether you survived or thrived. Things haven't changed much. The more educated, loved, rich, or famous—the more important you are—the more opportunities you have and the lower your risk of danger. This is why the emotional center has so much control over behavior. The monkey remembers when ostracization by the pack was a death sentence. This explains some very dark conundrums of human nature. That some people remain in clearly abusive relationships can be explained by the biological, inherited survival instinct for tribe and home. To strike out into the unknown takes a feat of courage that is often misunderstood. It must take a momentous force of will for an adolescent girl to run away from home alone with no backup system in place, or for a battered woman to pull up the only roots she has, risk ostracization from family and friends, and move her children to the street or a shelter. Like the lizard, the monkey is not concerned with quality of life, just survival and replication. The monkey says home is safest, even when that's not the case.

As much as we like to think we are rational, thoughtful beings, we all have an identity, a personal story that lives largely in our monkey brain. Anytime that belief system is threatened, the monkey's hackles go up. The monkey's high concern for brand names, ego, identity, and social status causes quite a few woes: conservative, liberal, Christian, Muslim, Jewish, black, white, straight, trans. This is where knee-jerk reactions cause us to work against our own best interests and even put us in danger. The monkey brain feels intensely logical, even as our cognitive faculties are mostly offline. Dr. Drew Westen, author of *The Political Brain*, points out that when we defend our beliefs and political views, we feel entirely rational, but in functional magnetic resonance images (FMRIs) most of the activity is in the limbic system.[7] The monkey brain.

> *The Monkey cannot distinguish between humiliation and death…. Soldiers could not be relied on in wartime if the fear of being laughed at as a coward didn't override the fear of death.*
> —Rory Miller, author, conflict analyst

The human brain is the part most concerned with well-being. As the seat of self-observation and analytical thinking, it is tasked with monitoring and managing the lizard and monkey. This newest brain offers the tools we need to stop the monkey from repeating the same argument of twenty years with Mom—it's where we can ask, is this a means to an end, or is my monkey repeating this social script because it is addictively satisfying and confirms the dependability of this relationship? The logical human brain is where we can spot and disarm social scripts that cause us to make accusations, justifications, and dangerous decisions based entirely on emotion.

> *If you feel emotion, if you are passionate about your cause, the part of your brain that makes good decisions is offline.*
> —Rory Miller, author, conflict analyst

Flip the Script

Social scripts exist to keep groups together if not individually satisfied. In early human social life, people lived within tribes or villages and knew the inhabitants their whole lives. While our modern daily lives have become exponentially more complex, neither the core social issues nor the methods we employ for dealing with them have changed very much.

---

[7] "Emory Study Lights Up the Political Brain," *ScienceDaily*, January 6, 2006, https://www.sciencedaily.com/releases/2006/01/060131092225.htm.

In his book *Conflict Communication*, Rory Miller lists the types of issues common social scripts evolved to navigate:
- to create and maintain a social group (couple, family, team)
- to establish and maintain a hierarchy
- to enforce mores—the how, when, and why things are done the way they are

It is not the goal of this book to describe these processes in depth. But it is helpful to understand the basics of why we repeat behaviors so that we can take steps to avoid the unproductive or harmful ones.

Most human interactions run the same scripts over and over: one-upmanship, who's right, who chooses the movie tonight, why does he have more than I do? Scripts are powerful and quicker than conscious thought. It takes practice recognizing them and breaking their hold, but recognizing your own scripts helps you recognize other people's.

It's early. You're first to the office as usual. You settle with your coffee just as your ex-boyfriend walks in and begins begging you to come back. You remember that he knows your schedule, which hasn't changed in years. You wish you'd done something about that—maybe locked the office door until 9 am. He becomes increasingly acrimonious. You hope someone will come in, and soon. You've seen this behavior in small moments—he knows just how to push until you lose your temper—but something is off this time. You forget the danger, you've had it, you won't be cowed on your own turf! You put your hands on your hips and tell him what you really think of him.

Does your final release of anger accomplish anything? Do you feel better afterward or does an unstable person with nothing to lose get physical?

I knew a woman who ended up in a coma after a similar incident.

We've all felt the need to get the last word in even when there is nothing to be gained and plenty to lose. The last word is a powerful monkey script. It means, I won this round. Even when you didn't. That feeling keeps us on script despite very loud warnings from the human brain that we are headed over the falls.

The monkey is full of big emotions, and it seems that the stronger we feel about a thing, the less we are thinking to logical and effective

Chapter 2: Me, Myself, and Conflict

ends. Miller writes, "If you feel emotion, if you are passionate about your cause, the part of your brain that makes good decisions is off-line." Once triggered, the limbic system can create a chain reaction; one person triggers another. This is one reason people who remain calm when others are triggered tend to impress or unnerve us.

Here are some steps to recognizing and hacking an ineffective script:

- Since high emotion is key, we might try to be aware of our own emotional states and the physical sensations that go along with charged emotions. These are different for everyone and require a special sort of self-awareness. Stay alert for that burn in your chest, the tightness in your temples, the ring in your ears, the dryness in your throat, the butterflies in your stomach, the cascade of thoughtless words that signify highly emotional states and behavior traps.
- As soon as you realize emotion is at the wheel, you must first and foremost de-escalate yourself. To this end you might take a breather. Conscious breathing helps with de-escalation partly because it causes you to focus on something else, but it also activates the vagus nerve, which regulates the parasympathetic nervous system. Exhaling twice as long as inhaling is one simple formula—that's a two-count inhale to a four-count exhale, or a three-count to a six-count, and so on. A breath or pause before talking may also help to keep words from slipping out before they get permission.

  For many people, pausing or breathing during an emotional moment can be almost physically painful. The urge to speak can have a similar flavor and even pathology as the urge to gamble or light up a cigarette. Stopping yourself from rolling down an emotional hill may cause extreme psychological discomfort and takes practice.

- Pausing keeps you from getting into trouble, but it is also an opportunity to gather information. Active listening is one of the most powerful tools for script change. High emotions block the ability to listen heartfully. Often there are words in our minds and mouths before we have even processed what someone has said. Pausing to listen allows others to feel heard and also offers the opportunity to find points of mutual connection. There is also a tactical and practical advantage in knowing more about the other person than they know about you.

Habit 5: Seek first to understand, then to be understood. Influence others by developing a deep understanding of their needs and perspectives.
—Stephen Covey, *The 7 Habits of Highly Effective People*

What is sama?
Sama is deep listening.
Sama is whirling dance....
Intelligence is a tree.
In sama, you hear the breeze in its branches
You hear the branches bloom.
Listen to the musicians.
Listen with your heart.
Listen with your skin.
Doors open.
—Rumi, 13th century Sufi poet

As soon as you determine that you are running an ineffective script, your options are:

- to stay on script, which means you are accepting the trajectory or consequences of the script. If a certain script is expected and pacifying, it may be better to let it play out
- or you can flip the script by changing your role. You might try reframing your viewpoint and approaching the situation differently. This is especially difficult when opinions are polarized: between teenagers and parents or teachers, between people on different sides of the gender discussion, or between those of different cultural, political, or religious views. As a parent, I can approach my son as the boss or I can meet him as a coach. I can insist he do things my way, or I can show curiosity and help him learn to solve his own problems. Each of these roles will run

different scripts and drastically change the outcome of an interaction (and ultimately a relationship).

Flipping a script requires us to tap into a different part of ourselves while we are already processing emotionally strenuous data. Actors practiced at sliding into different roles have experience with this. The rest of us are so egocentric that changing our role even a bit can feel like a kind of betrayal of self. This is of course emotional and not logical.

You may be able to reframe and flip the script by finding common ground. When you find that someone you have always disagreed with about politics and labeled one of the bad guys turns out to know more about curing your devastating cluster headaches than any doctor you've ever met, it opens new lines of communication. Finding something of value vastly increases your chances of connection. And almost every human being has something of value to offer. That hardly matters if they pose an imminent threat, but there are many smaller life-altering interactions that can be managed this way.

You might also choose to reset the interaction with a tactical apology; say out loud, as much to yourself as the other guy, "Sorry, I got a bit too emotional there, let's start over."

- You also have the option of rejecting a script altogether by ending the interaction. This can make things better or worse, depending on the situation. You might even point the script out to the other person, but it won't always be well-received. It may bring the person's attention to a lack of effectiveness or it may feel like a show of superiority. Sometimes it stops the script in its tracks, sometimes it raises hackles. Choose wisely.

One may understand the cosmos, but never the ego; the self is more distant than any star.
 —G.K. Chesterton, *The Logic of Elfland,*
    Orthodoxy 1908

Mind-Setting Part 1

> *We are all born with a brain, but no one supplies a manual.*
> —Karim Hajee, life coach, author

In cognitive psychology, mindset is a group of attitudes relating to and stemming from beliefs, principles, ethics, morals, values, life experience, personal philosophy, culture, disposition, emotional makeup, and current life context, among other things. It's a complex discussion, and it's important not to feel helpless and accept your mindset as unchangeable. Your mindset at any given time is not simply a product of what happened that day or that week, nor is it an immutable result of the way you were raised—it is within your control to a significant degree.

My good friend Karim Hajee once told me that we are all born with a brain, yet no one ever gives us a manual. No one ever sits us down and explains how our brain works. It's like hopping in the car and figuring out how to drive on the highway. We learn what we learn and miss a lot. We get lazy and don't use all our mental tools. The older we get, the more set in our ways we become and the more difficult it is to make changes to our respective operating manuals.

The emotional and logical areas of our brain work as a system of checks and balances. Discerning which is at work at any given time arms us with the flexibility to make effective choices. All our mechanisms and parts have roles to play. Like an orchestra, too much of one sound or another creates dissonance.

Learn about your mindset through observation. Make no judgements. Are you in a proactive or reactive state? Are you aware of what is driving your current mindset? Would you know how to change it? Strive gently to become an impartial, nonjudgmental observer of your own mind and cultivate the ability to make suggestions and adjustments to the way you feel about any particular situation.

We will revisit mindset throughout this book.

Awareness Part 1: Pay Attention!

> *You see but you do not observe.*
> —Sir Arthur Conan Doyle, *Sherlock Holmes*

We hear a lot about awareness. We are told to "pay attention!" by parents, teachers, and even strangers on the subway. But what is awareness? How does it work? Where is our roadmap for how to manage our attention in daily life? We'll talk a lot about self-awareness or internal awareness in this book, but external awareness or awareness of situation, environment, and your place within them is multi-faceted and multi-sensory and improves through the building and cultivation of the multiple "muscles" of awareness, attention, and observation.

Overall, living in predominantly safe societies has domesticated us. We live in "a vacation state of mind," as park ranger Debo Cox says in Laurence Gonzales's book *Everyday Survival*. We worry a lot, but about the wrong things. We are blinded by boredom, laziness, and overstimulation from electronic devices among other things, and our attention spans are decreasing by the minute and the generation. Our brains cannot process every bit of the internal and external information—thoughts, sights, sounds, memories, emotions—it is bombarded with; it must make choices. Those choices amount to what we call attention. In her brilliant book, *Visual Intelligence,* Amy E. Herman writes, "Today, more people have access to cell phones than to working toilets." She continues by telling us that a 2005 study at King's College at London University found that distracted workers suffered a 10- to 15-point IQ loss—a greater loss than comes from using marijuana, and one that brings an adult male down to the IQ level of an eight-year-old child.

There are different types or levels of awareness and attention. We spend much of our lives on autopilot in familiar environments and have preexisting expectations of how things will go. Active awareness gets turned on when things are different or something alerts us. Hypervigilance is a state of sensory sensitivity in which the nervous system is overreactive and views normal information about the environment as potentially threatening. This is a common nervous system adaptation to

PTSD and trauma and causes inappropriate and exaggerated responses that block normal processing of environmental information (which makes managing hypervigilance highly important to safety and the practice of protective offense—more about PTSD in chapter 10).

But where do we put our brains in daily life?

You are probably familiar with Jeff Cooper's Color Codes, which provide a framework for situational awareness by using colors to describe levels of awareness and readiness in potentially dangerous situations. Cooper was a lieutenant colonel in the Marines, but he also taught high school and college history. Cooper developed his Color Codes because he felt the weapon and even the skills a person carried with them were less important than their mindset. He used his model to illustrate how different mindsets affect a person's ability to survive a lethal encounter. Though some may dismiss Cooper's useful model as some clunky government method of alerting the public, it is a simple way to determine where your mind should be at any given moment, especially when intuition whispers in your ear.

According to Cooper, when we zone out, we are in a white awareness mindset, unprepared for adversity, and therefore vulnerable to sudden changes in our environment. Yellow illustrates a state of relaxed alertness in which we are aware of our surroundings. Orange puts us in a state of alert over a potential emergency and causes us to actively seek more information. Red (sometimes black) is full alert as in exiting a burning building or actively fighting for our lives.

The colors don't really matter—the concept does. Being entirely off guard should be reserved for rest and sleep. Consider spending most of your time in yellow, or relaxed alert. Cultivating a state of general relaxed awareness and choosing to live there can be empowering.

For another awareness model, look no further than thousands of years of Buddhist teachings. A standard message in Buddhism is to live mindfully in the present. This internal state keeps us interacting with ourselves and our environment in real time. Easier said than done. Modern life is relentless, but rather than perfection, the goal is to gently nudge ourselves when we zone out in public, to be mindful and aware of mental processes in real time, to worry less about past or future. When we find ourselves obsessing over things we have no control over, or dwelling on where we might be in the future, we can try to come back to where we are now.

Author and firearms instructor Kathy Jackson lines trainees up and runs them through some drills. Students remove their guns from their holsters and pause in a low ready position, looking once over each shoulder as instructed; they then stretch their weapons out in front of them into isosceles position, aim at the target, and pull the trigger slowly, twice. Once they complete the drill and methodically reholster, Kathy asks everyone what they saw behind them. No one answers. No one remembers seeing anything. After she points this out, no one misses the opportunity to name the details of what was behind them for the rest of the day.

How does all this play into a protective mindset? When you live in the present moment, you walk differently, your head is up, your eyes are moving, and you notice more. When you are aware of yourself and your surroundings, you don't look like prey. This is an excellent mindset in general, but it is also the best mindset for avoiding danger. I was a bully magnet in my early school years, but as soon as I began taking martial arts, I also began walking different and taking up more space. And like a switch being flipped, the bullying stopped. An important side effect of relaxed awareness is how well it works to remove you from the criminal radar.

Recap

- The Circle of Concern represents everything we dwell on, fuss over, and worry about; the Circle of Influence represents things we actually have control over.
- Conflict is unavoidable and necessary; conflict management tools include self-awareness, recognizing, reappraising, and reframing.
- Recognize the early signs of stress.
- The way we think about stress may be worse than the stress itself. Reappraise stress as excitement or something more beneficial to your nervous system.
- Reframe stressful situations by considering other viewpoints or channeling someone you respect.
- The triune brain theory is a model for understanding our reactions and responses.

- o The Lizard Brain (basal ganglia) is the oldest, most survival-centric part of the brain and most resistant to change.
- o The Monkey Brain (limbic system) is the social-emotional center, focused on identity, and social status. It causes us to feel we are being logical, even when we are not.
- o The Human Brain (neocortex) is the seat of self-observation and analytical thinking. It monitors and balances the lizard and monkey.

- Miller says common social scripts evolved to:

  o create and maintain the social group (couple, family, team)
  o to establish and maintain the hierarchy
  o to enforce mores

- Script-hacking is one of the most effective yet underrated self-defense techniques, and recognizing your own scripts helps you see other people's scripts.
- Steps to recognizing and hacking an ineffective script:
  - o Recognize when your monkey is driving your responses (don't deny it). Become aware of your emotional states and the physical sensations that go along with them.
  - o As soon as you realize emotion is at the wheel, you must first and foremost de-escalate yourself.
    - Take a breath. Breathe deliberately and create a moment of pause. Pausing keeps you from getting into trouble, but it is also an opportunity to gather information.
    - Active listening is one of the most powerful tools for script change and opportunity to gather information.
- As soon as you determine that a script is ineffective or even dangerous, your options are to:
  - o Stay on script: this means you are accepting the trajectory or consequences of the script. If a certain script is expected and pacifying, it may be better to let it play out.
  - o Flip the script and change the outcome:
    - Try to find common ground.
    - Try to reset the interaction with a tactical apology; say out loud, as much to yourself as the other guy, "Sorry, I got a bit too emotional there, let's start over."

o Reject the script by ending the interaction or by pointing the script out to the other party.
- Become an impartial, nonjudgmental observer of your own mind.
- Living in predominantly safe societies has domesticated us. We worry a lot but about the wrong things. Use a simple model like the Cooper Color Codes or look to Buddhist philosophy to help you discover ways to cultivate "mindfulness" and stay present and aware of the world around you so you don't look like prey.

Suggested Practices

 "Begin with the end in mind" as Stephen Covey says. What do you want to get out of protective-offense training? Be specific. Make a list in your journal. Revisit and revise.

 If you were a superhero, what would your powers be? Make a list of traits you would like to have. Don't just choose the obvious ones; be creative and have fun.

 Observe yourself in conflict then write about it in your journal. How do you respond to adversity in general? Anger? Frustration? Sadness? Are there specific steps you usually go through before things get better? Do you get quiet and hold it in? Freak out? Are you fair to other people? Is your temper short? Are you passive-aggressive? What would those closest to you say? Be honest with yourself.

 Write about what unnerves, worries, or scares you. Persistent concerns keep our minds busy and distracted. Write in your journal about what itches at the back of your mind or wakes you up at night. This may take more than one session. Is there a common denominator? Could all your fears be attributed to one or two issues? Understanding your worries and fears opens up a conversation and helps you clarify what is within your circle of influence. Be kind to yourself and your students if you try this. Anger about fear only intensifies fear.

 Take the red pill: Remember this from *The Matrix*? Take the blue pill and you stay in your comfort zone where you know the rules. Take the red pill and your reality changes drastically.

Practice discomfort once a month, once a week, or even once a day. Make the most difficult task of the day the first thing you do. Fear of speaking? Practice in front of a mirror and stand up at the next PTA meeting. A food you refuse to try? Clear your mind of preconceived ideas.

Getting out of your comfort zone forces exploration and banishes complacency. This may mean doing something emotional that has been a sticking point for you: apologizing to someone you've been meaning to apologize to, or talking to your boss about your future (make sure to pick the best time for the boss, not just for you). Pick something that is nagging at you today—and do it. Make discomfort comfortable (always do your research or take someone experienced—and fun—with you when trying new, potentially dangerous activities). Try skydiving, learn to swim, join a polar bear club and jump in the icy lake (after obtaining permission from your doctor).

Push your envelope gently and intelligently. Who could you be without your own self-imposed restraints? A person who gets the tough stuff done without hesitation? A person who makes decisions and carries them out without complaint?

Often, the most disastrous thing you can do in a self-defense situation is nothing. When we spend too much time in our comfort zones, we become complacent and the muscles responsible for quick, decisive actions atrophy. Decisively facing stressful circumstances forces the mind to expand, to troubleshoot, to engage in the highest forms of learning. Exercise your mental reflexes. Being the first one to do the tough job without complaint, to attack fears without hesitation, and to solve problems no one else wants to is a low-level superpower. We are calling Take the Red Pill an exercise, but really we want it to become a habit.

CHAPTER 3

Where Wolf?

Inga: "Werewolf!"
Dr. Frankenstein: "Werewolf?"
Igor: "There wolf. There castle."
　　—*Young Frankenstein*, film by Mel Brooks

We like to talk big, vampires do. "I'm going to destroy the world," that's just tough guy talk. Strutting around with your friends over a pint of blood. The truth is, I like this world. You've got dog racing. Manchester United. And you've got people, billions of people, walking around like Happy Meals with legs…
　　—Spike from *Buffy the Vampire Slayer*, TV show

Criminals and devious people often live out of sight, out of mind. The domestic and wild universes coexist the way flying insects coexist with aquatic life, but every now and then an insect flies too close to the water's surface and something hungry jumps out.

Criminals are aware of the domestic universe (it is their job), but the knowledge does not go the other way. They watch while we walk around—as Spike from *Buffy the Vampire Slayer* says, "Like Happy Meals with legs." It's our job to seek answers, not the world's job to make things easy for us.

What if there were no right or wrong, only the simplest way to get what you needed? You could choose to accomplish things in a timely manner, without concern for rules, even if it caused trouble for someone else.

For some people, manipulation and abuse are useful tools. The long, slow way to a goal may ultimately win friends and influence people, but it generally isn't the fastest method. Most people choose diplomacy over violence because of a built-in social switch that says we need one another and it feels bad to hurt others or because diplomacy is ultimately safer and leads to longer-lasting results. Not everyone follows these rules. Diversity is important to lifeforms of all types for many reasons. A thankfully small percentage of people have talents (manipulation, slight-of-hand-or-word) that they use to acquire or do things that are beneficial to them and detrimental to others. They don't feel guilty about their methods, and they may even see you as a weak link begging to be taken advantage of. They keep us on our toes, or we lose our toes.

He's manipulative, she's narcissistic, they're abusive—at what point does a relationship veer from problematic to dangerous? How do you recognize when a line has been crossed? What are your choices? All this begins with a foray into the minds of those we consider troublemakers.

Acceptance and Pragmatism

> *It is difficult to believe and accept that anyone we like and identify with is capable of [horrific] acts against their fellow human beings.... This simple naive tendency is possibly, more than any other factor, responsible for the perpetuation of atrocity and horror in our world today.*
>
> —Lt. Col Dave Grossman, former West Point psychology professor, Army Ranger, author

Chapter 3: Where Wolf?

Criminals and deviant personalities are part of our world. We can no sooner purge the planet of them than eliminate a single gas from the atmosphere. To expect the police to be everywhere at once would be unrealistic to a fault. Society is controlled chaos.

Each of us possesses the ability to attract or repel predators. What we don't know can hurt us. We are rightly on guard when situations and behaviors are unfamiliar, but we may be more at risk from situations that mimic ones we are familiar with or that change under our radar. A familiar scenario lulls us into complacency. By the time we realize there's a gap—that the boss is not the decent person we assumed, that we are in a relationship with someone capable of sociopathic behavior—the sinkhole has opened and is swallowing us whole.

We must recognize and accept the existence of predators. If we busy ourselves questioning why, or blaming society, we will ask the wrong questions. Criminals are part of our world. We can ignore them or function under the delusion that society should create a buffer between us and them. But the fact is society can only intervene once something has gone wrong.

We evolved in tribes because we were stronger that way. Those who excelled athletically could climb higher trees to gain access to food or a better view of the surroundings. Those inclined to nurturing and healing had a job, as did those who were natural storytellers or entertainers. More people meant more diverse resources, abilities, and knowledge. So, the concepts of fair play, rules, and trust evolved along with social relationships.

There will always be someone who seeks to circumvent the system, whose brain is wired differently, or whose original tribe didn't pass down the social rules. Deviant behavior wins the practitioner whatever they seek: money, power, sex, excitement, resources. In most cases, the ultimate result is banishment from the group—divorce, prison, or worse. In thankfully rare instances, the deviant behavior enjoys continuous success. So long as it is successful, it is likely to continue.

More than two thousand years ago, Sun Tzu said, "If you know your enemy and yourself, you will not be imperiled in a hundred battles." You may have heard it rephrased to fit neatly into a business meeting: "In order to succeed you must know yourself *and* your enemy." Gavin de Becker, author of *The Gift of Fear,* says, "The importance of seeing things from the perspective of the person whose behavior you are predicting cannot be overstated." So, it seems the experts agree.

Common Ground

> *I used to tell my rookies that every one of our inmates was three people: the person who did the crime; the person we had in custody; and the person their family knew.*
> —Rory Miller, author, conflict analyst

It isn't necessary to empathize with criminals to understand the way they think and function, but when we see criminals as utterly unlike us, we blind ourselves. We say, "He came out of nowhere" and "There was nothing I could have done" when we may simply have missed the signs.

Often, the line between criminal behavior and average behavior is more quantitative than qualitative; it's not so much that a criminal will do something you wouldn't, it's that he will take it further than you would. You might have shoplifted; you are less likely to have robbed a bank.

Cognitive bias refers to a method of information processing that relies on an individual's subjective construct of reality rather than objective input. This form of processing circumvents the need for new constructs of common circumstances and creates thought shortcuts. However, if the construct is inaccurate, so are all the resulting calculations.

We all rationalize and lie on occasion based on our perception of the facts and our respective cognitive biases. We begin as children who see the world as we are, not as it is. A child's brain is singularly focused on navigating her world and bending it to her will. Children seek loopholes and creative ways of gaining control. It's their job to bend rules, sometimes to breaking. Most of us eventually learn new methods, but if childhood strategies are successful and encouraged, or trauma interrupts brain growth, the behavior may persist into adulthood. The result is a person who lacks the capacity for complex social interactions and methods of problem solving. Children and criminals often both use the loudest or most destructive behavior to get their way. As Abraham Maslow said in 1966, "I suppose it is tempting, if the only tool you have is a hammer, to treat everything as if it were a nail." We all forget to bring our tools every now and then; some people only have the one.

Human beings are pros at blocking, deflecting, reframing, and rationalizing to turn things to their advantage or make themselves look or feel better. These adaptations often help us survive by pushing us to become stronger, smarter, or more important. Occasionally, they get in our way. Even helpful adaptations can become bad habits when overused.

Most criminals and devious people don't consider themselves to be such. Common rationalizations might include thinking you're smarter or more talented than someone else and deserve more or that you're evening an unfair playing field or looking out for yourself rather than taking anything away from anyone.

Even on our best behavior, most of us have broken a few laws—run a red light or stop sign at the very least. Did you tell the officer that you didn't see it even though you did? That the light was yellow when you went you went through? Did you rationalize by telling yourself the officer was mean and didn't deserve to be right, or that you're basically a good person?

There are different types of understanding, and sometimes creating parallels within our own experience can provide a deeper grasp of knowledge—a feeling, rather than just a knowing. And when you're trying to avoid danger, the lizard and monkey are faster than the human. When we admit we are all devious thinkers some of the time, we may find dodgy behaviors easier to spot.

> *There's a critically important point to understand about violent people. They are trapped in a world that is all about them. All the average person sees is the violence. What you don't see is the intense self-loathing, chronic anger, warped perceptions, fear, paranoia, blaming behavior, and other demons that drive these people. And the reason you don't see this is because they are either deeply hidden beneath layers upon layers of rationalization, or because, at ground zero, you're too busy experiencing the blast to see it clearly.*
> —Marc MacYoung, author, conflict analyst, expert witness

Scary People

We gathered at the window to watch the crowd form as police tied off the street in front of my building with yellow tape. I never had to go anywhere; all I had to do was look out the window of my historic East Village block and something interesting, political, momentous even, seemed to be taking place. This was new, though.

The police discreetly searched a pile of garbage bags that had accumulated due to the garbage strike. They loaded a few into a van and shouted at the crowd to back up. I wondered what on earth was in the garbage that was so fascinating.

Later that night, the navy-blue sedans pulled up. Two men in suits stepped out, climbed the stairs, and rang our bell. Flashing a badge, one of them said someone was murdered. MURDERED! Did we know a guy named Milan Viertl? My mother had nicknamed him Milano nearly twenty years earlier when he emigrated from Czechoslovakia.

"Yes…?"

"How well?"

"Twenty years well. He's family. He and my daughter share a birthday."

"When was the last time you saw him?"

"A few days ago, Thursday—no, Wednesday. Why? Is he in trouble?"

"There was a murder. We think it's him."

My mother snorted, "No, Milano couldn't hurt a fly."

"No, we think it's him in the bags."

My vision blurred.

"It would have happened Wednesday."

My mother stammered. "The new roommate, I forget his name, said Milano was in the shower." Her eyes glazed, a kind of shock. She spoke in a smaller voice and sat involuntarily. I followed. "Milano doesn't have a shower."

I didn't have to turn to look at our old tenement tub in the kitchen.

Milano was annoying. He was a big personality, loud, older than me by fifteen years. He invited himself over to dinner often, and he liked to scare me when I was little by growling at the door to be let in. He would do anything to annoy me. Neighbors called him my big brother.

Chapter 3: Where Wolf?

My mother testified. Later she identified the body (Milan hadn't seen his family in many years) and organized the wake.

Before they left, I mumbled to the navy-suited men that it didn't make sense to leave evidence so close to home. They told me, contrary to popular knowledge, most murderers aren't all that careful. It's not uncommon for criminals to hide evidence close to the scene if its difficult to dispose of. No one has a car in New York, cabbies won't pick you up with trash bags, a wheelbarrow would be suspicious.

If it weren't for the garbage strike, my friend would have simply disappeared.

Thankfully, my experience is not the norm. Though those unfettered by the social rules the rest of us follow have an edge, most people are not murderers. I do wonder, though, how things might have gone had my friend identified the early signs that his roommate was dangerous.

Scary people exist. Your job is to know what to look for and to put the pieces together before these people become your problem. This, more than anything, is the goal of this book, because getting out of trouble is always messier than staying out.

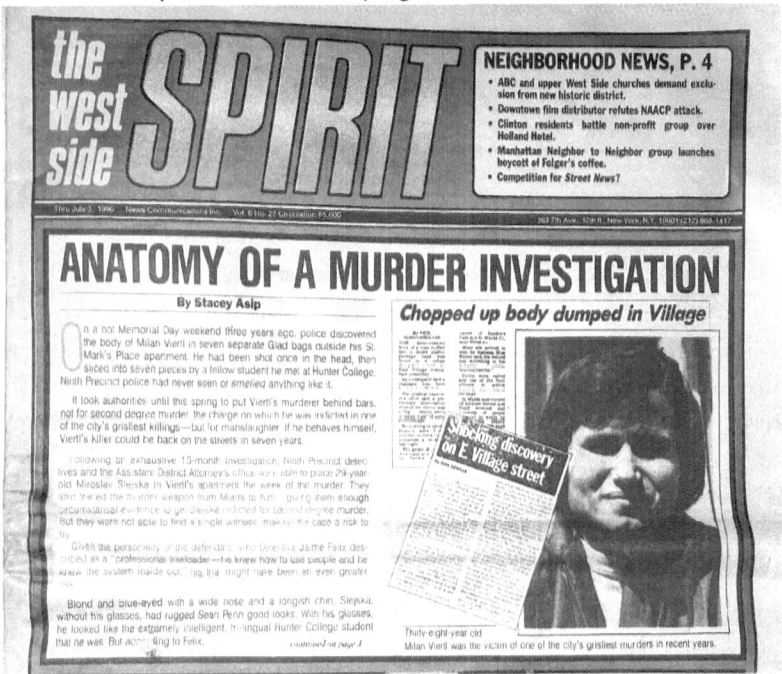

July 1990 *The West Side Spirit* newspaper

Sociopaths and psychopaths are all the rage on TV. They usually show up as one of two types: quiet and meticulous or unstrung. In reality, they may appear more normal than we would like. There is some confusion about whether sociopathy and psychopathy are different conditions or basically the same. Dr. Scott Bonn, author of *Why We Love Serial Killers: The Curious Appeal of the World's Savage Murderers*, contends that sociopathy is a learned behavior resulting from "nurture" and psychopathy is the result of a genetic underdevelopment of the emotional and impulse centers of the brain. Opinions vary. Luckily, we don't need to differentiate between the two to understand important aspects of both behavior patterns.

We can think of sociopathy and psychopathy as personality disorders characterized by a distinct lack of conscience and empathy, inability to make meaningful connections with others, and generally opportunistic, antisocial, or narcissistic traits which only, on rare occasions, are accompanied by violent tendencies. The statistic used in *The Sociopath Next Door* by Martha Stout, PhD, say roughly one in twenty-five people lacks what we call conscience.

> *I don't feel guilty for anything.*
> *I feel sorry for people who feel guilt.*
>   —Ted Bundy

Scientifically, we are usually referring to one of two personality disorders: narcissistic personality disorder (NPD) or antisocial personality disorder (ASPD or APD), cluster-B personality disorders as categorized by the *Diagnostic and Statistical Manual of Mental Disorders* (DSM-V). While both NPD and ASPD are marked by a lack of empathy and manipulative tendencies, NPD is characterized by a need for admiration and a grandiose sense of self-importance whereas ASPD leans toward a disregard for social norms and a history of criminal behavior or conduct disorders in childhood. But perhaps a more useful way to recognize these personality types is in the context of affordances.

Psychologist James J. Gibson coined the term affordances in 1966 to describe the possible actions that an environment or object offers an individual. Where one person may see another as a neighbor, friend, or coworker, another may instead perceive a *thing*—a walking ATM, for instance, or a toy. There are times even you might think this way; for instance, in the moment you are drowning, you might see someone who jumps in to save you as a floatation device and inadvertently pull them under. So, a key aspect of the conditions we call sociopathy and psychopathy might, in pragmatic terms, be the tendency to see other people primarily as resources.

If you spend time with children, you know they can rationalize anything. They can stand there with crumbs on their faces, swear they didn't eat the last cookie, be shocked at your accusations, and even retaliate for your cruelty. They are 100-percent certain they are in the right. They will grow out of it, though, whereas adult sociopaths are unlikely to. This simple reframing exercise is one way to make sure we don't see criminals as so foreign that we forget they are people whose behavior we can understand and therefore predict.

Conscienceless people are often the life of the party. They take pleasure in manipulation, and the best tool to this end is charm. If you can get people to trust you, the sky is the limit. They put on a show of emotion so they can live in the world and avoid being labeled and separated from their prime resource.

There are many reasons for deviant and criminal behavior but it isn't necessary to dissect them here. Mental illness, drug use, and socioeconomics are all connected and play various roles. But the signs of potentially violent behavior are similar and therefore recognizable with training.

> *To charm is to compel, to control by allure or attraction. Think of charm as a verb, not a trait. If you consciously tell yourself, "This person is trying to charm me" as opposed to, "This person is charming," you'll be able to see around it.*
> —Gavin de Becker, author of *The Gift of Fear*

Concepts and Models

Whether violent or merely manipulative, learning to avoid relationships with dangerous or conscienceless people plays an important part in any self-defense regimen. Dr. Robert Hare, a professor of psychology and renowned expert on psychopathy, recommends understanding how to spot these toxic individuals as the only course to avoidance and safety. Hare developed the Psychopathy Checklist, a list of personality traits to watch for.[8]

Hare's Traits from the Psychopathy Checklist (abridged):
- lack of sincerity, remorse, guilt, or empathy
- superficial charm
- grandiose sense of self-worth
- prone to boredom, craving wild stimulation in the form of sex, crime, and sometimes violence
- use of pathological deception, often with a carefully calculated goal
- parasitic lifestyle—living off others
- poor behavioral control in the form of sudden outbursts of anger or impulsivity
- history of promiscuity or series of short relationships (easily bored)
- problems with rules and authority, history of childhood behavioral problems, impulsivity, or juvenile delinquency
- lack of realistic long-term goals, general irresponsibility
- failure to accept responsibility for own actions (blame always lies elsewhere)

Many people have one or two of these traits—everyone is impulsive and self-centered on occasion or may live off a parent or spouse for short periods—but a combination of these traits should raise a red flag. Knowing yourself is just as important as knowing others. If you like to fix or nurture people, be especially wary—sociopaths may hone in on you. A friend might need a place to stay and never leave. She may claim to have been the victim of a financial scam, pull you down her rabbit hole, and rob you of your emotional and financial resources. Always remember that a solid, self-aware friend would never put their needs over yours—would never insist you share their pain.

If you notice that a person in your social circle exhibits more than one of the traits on Hare's checklist on an ongoing basis, you may want to limit your exposure. Hopefully, you'll spot the signs well before the wedding.

---

8 Robert D. Hare, "Hare Psychopathy Checklist–Revised," https://criminologyweb.com/wp-content/uploads/2019/12/Hare-Psychopathy-Checklist-Revised-PCLR.pdf.

Chapter 3: Where Wolf?

Should you fall in love with me due to my
relentless charm assault, that's okay too.
—Martin Short, *Only Murders in the Building*
(TV show)

Dr. Martha Stout, who wrote *The Sociopath Next Door* and *Outsmarting the Sociopath Next Door*, says we are all likely to deal with a sociopath or two at some point in our lives. Here is her take on dealing with sociopaths and the like.

Stout's Thirteen Rules for Dealing with Sociopaths in Everyday Life:[9]

1. **Accept that conscienceless people exist** and that they often look just like us rather than like the monsters we expect.
2. **Don't let authority or impressive labels fool you.** Doctors, educators, and leaders of all kinds may also be sociopaths. Always heed your intuition.
3. **Observe the Rule of Three when embarking on a new relationship** of any kind: one lie, one broken promise, one neglected responsibility may be a misunderstanding, two may be a serious error in judgment, but three is a habit, and deceit is a benchmark behavior of conscienceless people. Don't share your life, work, money, or secrets with this person.
4. **Question authority,** especially when everyone around you is drinking the Kool-Aid. Remember Stanley Milgram's famous experiment on obedience to authority and never follow orders blindly.
5. **Suspect flattery.** Always look for the man behind the curtain. Is there an ulterior motive or intent to manipulate?
6. **Don't mistake fear for respect.** They are never the same thing.
7. **Don't play the game.** Stout says, "Intrigue is a sociopath's tool… Resist the temptation to compete… outsmart, psychoanalyze, or even banter…" Don't allow yourself to be seduced by the game only to find out you are trapped.
8. **The best way to protect yourself is by avoidance.** Since sociopaths exist outside the social contract, including them in social relationships comes at high risk. Excluding them will not hurt

---

[9] Lanre Dahunsi, "Martha Stout's Thirteen Rules for Dealing with Sociopaths in Everyday Life," lanredahunsi.com, July 23, 2021, https://www.lanredahunsi.com/martha-stouts-thirteen-rules-for-dealing-with-sociopaths-in-everyday-life/.

their feelings though they may try to make you feel as though you have deeply injured them.
9. **Question your automatic tendency to be sympathetic.** In polite society, empathy and sympathy are reflexive. A sociopath will take advantage of this for exploitive purposes. Opt for avoidance or assertiveness. Stout says, "Do not be afraid to be unsmiling and calmly to the point."
10. **Do not try to redeem the unredeemable.** We must embody the disappointing life lesson that, even with the best intentions, we cannot control or alter another person's behavior or character. Stout says, "Avoid the irony of becoming caught up in the same ambition he has—to control."
11. **Never agree to help a sociopath conceal their true nature.** Stout says, "'Please don't tell,' said tearfully, is the trademark plea of thieves, child abusers, and sociopaths." Ask yourself if a thief deserves your help more than others deserve to be warned. "You owe me" is another trademark demand.
12. **Define your own psyche.** Don't allow anyone to convince you to be like them or that society is a useless construct. The only way society works is if we are all willing to share resources, including emotional ones like trust.
13. **Living well is the best revenge.**

Dr. Stanton Samenow, who wrote a well-respected book on violence called *Inside the Criminal Mind,* posits that a criminal's needs at any given moment can be more important than life itself; fairness, synergy, and compromise just don't factor into the final decision to engage in hurtful behavior. Armed with tools like The Psychopathy Checklist and The Thirteen Rules, we begin to form a picture of people to avoid using benchmarks we can recognize.

Statistics on mental illness and violence can be confusing. Mental illness is a sensitive subject, partly because some mentally ill people who become violent may only be trying to protect themselves from perceived danger rather than trying to cause harm.

I know a behaviorist who works with neurodiverse and mentally ill children. She once worked with a twelve-year-old boy who pulled a kitchen knife on her. He outweighed her by quite a bit. Thankfully,

Chapter 3: Where Wolf?

she had been trained and was able to talk him down. A close friend of mine has scars all over his arms where his daughter, who has autism, routinely bites and scratches him. It was not difficult for him to control her physically when she was eleven, but in puberty she shot up, and he's at a disadvantage since he's not willing to hurt her.

We should all be more open and empathetic in the presence of people suffering from emotional disorders, but we also need to protect ourselves and our children from dangerous behaviors regardless of the reasons. If you find yourself in a situation where you must interact with a distraught, confused, or desperate person, one thing is certain: do not escalate emotion.

Here are some thoughts from an article Rory Miller wrote as a corrections officer about dealing with criminal behavior in the mentally ill. Not all of what he wrote applies to a civilian situation, so I have extrapolated and paraphrased the parts that do. Always leave the area and get help if you feel you are in imminent danger.

Miller's Four A's for Dealing with Criminal Behavior in the Mentally Ill

- **Assume your assailant is intelligent**, even highly so, regardless of appearance or speech patterns. Never underestimate his intelligence—crazy does not mean stupid. Your attacker may see a hippo floating in the room, he may be high as the Empire State Building, but this doesn't preclude intelligence. He may be both nuts and smarter than you. If you assume you are smarter and it turns out you are incorrect, the decisions you make could be catastrophic.
- **Accept the reality of his experience.** The things that happen in his brain are just as real to him as the things happening in yours. That said, do not pretend to share the delusion. With few exceptions, most people in altered mental states have experience being there. Though the voices are real to him, he knows they are not real to you, and he may know you are lying. If he feels laughed at or condescended to, the situation may deteriorate quickly.
- **Access your calmest self.** There may be volatile mental and emotional factors that—along with drugs, alcohol, and the ups and down of adrenaline—don't play well together. If you are trying to de-escalate an increasingly agitated person, looking at the lower

face offers full attention without the challenge of direct eye contact. If you must speak, your voice should be slow, quiet, calm, and low-pitched. If you are not asked to speak, you feel you are in danger, and you can't leave, don't speak. Any movement should be smooth and slow. Do not touch him or invade his space. Do not try to control him or block exits. Avoid escalating emotion.

- **Actively listen and observe.** If something happened and you need to know what, or you are trying to assess his mental state, don't talk over him or make demands. If you speak at all, ask simple yes-or-no or close-ended questions. Never rush a stressed or impaired person since you might lose the chance to learn anything of value or, worse, cause an emotional break.

Social vs. Asocial Violence

Pleased to meet you, hope you guessed my name.
But what's puzzlin' you is the nature of my game.
—"Sympathy for the Devil," The Rolling Stones

Rory Miller and Marc MacYoung created the social/asocial designations that are central to an understanding of violent crime and to any program that purports to mitigate it.

Social violence occurs within a single species and involves familiar, socially acceptable ideas and goals. Common incidents of social aggression include bar fights over money, or women, or heated arguments at work over the chance to take charge of a project or team. Social violence also includes enforcing group rules within a family, school, gang, or other social group.

Social violence, like domestic violence, can go on for years, damage generations, and end in violence or murder. Hazing has killed university students in all kinds of bizarre ways, gang violence is notoriously horrific, and football (soccer) hooliganism is a well-documented phenomenon that involves groups of fans tearing through stadiums and neighborhoods destroying everything in their path and even killing.

Miller defines asocial violence as violence conducted against another species, or as if it were against another species, as in hunting or slaughtering. Othering is the process of perceiving other humans as alien and therefore unworthy of humane consideration. Miller says, "Asocial violence doesn't see the victim as a person but as an asset. In asocial violence the humanity of the victim does not enter the equation. An asocial predator will use more violence for less cause than a normal person." Asocial criminals are synonymous with sociopaths or psychopaths.

Miller urges that behavior that will deter a social predator may attract an asocial one. To a social individual, allowing a stranger to help you carry groceries to your car indicates that you're a trusting person who deserves consideration, while to an asocial person it's a green light to take advantage of you.

Within the asocial framework, we have another important delineation: *resource* versus *process violence*. An asocial resource predator attacks you for your wallet or your car—a resource; the resource is the goal. Mac Young also refers to these criminals as scavengers. An asocial process predator attacks you for the act of attacking; the act or process is the goal.

In resource violence the threat of violence is a tool to acquire a particular resource: wallet, jewelry, car. Violence isn't the goal because the threat alone often does the trick. In this case, you can sometimes give up the resource and be safe. The criminal might be clear about what he wants you to do, like put your wallet on the floor, or toss it too him gently. If the criminal is communicating with you, don't do anything to upset the delicate balance of adrenaline, like throw the wallet into the street. Professionals who regularly deal with criminals agree that you might push him to violence by pissing him off. He may not be averse to violence if you force his hand.

In asocial process violence, violence is the goal. This is the stuff of nightmares. You can't placate these people with things. This criminal will likely want to meet you at or move you to a private location, and you will need to think fast because the only reason for this is control. Don't believe him when he says he won't hurt you so long as you do what he says. Always listen to your intuition. Never let yourself be seduced by charm, power, or promises.

Behavior that will deter a social predator may attract an asocial one.
  —Rory Miller, author, conflict analyst

Recap

- Acceptance and pragmatism: criminals and deviant personalities are part of our world. When we question why, or blame others, we blind ourselves.
- Common ground: it's not so much that a criminal will do something you wouldn't, it's that he will take it further.
  o Humans use blocking, deflecting, and rationalizing to gain advantage. If strategies are successful or if trauma interrupts brain growth, the behaviors may persist, resulting in someone who lacks the capacity for complex social interactions and methods of problem-solving. When we admit we are all devious thinkers some of the time, we may find the behavior easier to recognize.
  o Cognitive bias is information processing that relies on an individual's subjective construct of reality rather than objective input. If the construct is inaccurate, so are all the resulting calculations.
- Scary people: NPD, ASPD, sociopathy, and psychopathy are personality disorders characterized by a distinct lack of conscience and empathy, inability to make meaningful connections, and general opportunistic traits which may on rare occasion be accompanied by violent tendencies.
- Concepts and models: armed with tools like Hare's Psychopathy Checklist and Stout's Thirteen Rules, we begin to form a picture of people to avoid using benchmarks we can recognize. Rory Miller's Four As give us ways to communicate with and de-escalate a potentially violent emotionally or mentally impaired person.
- Social VS asocial violence: Social violence occurs within a single species and involves familiar, socially accepted ideas and goals. Asocial violence has no familiar social goal. The target is othered and treated as nonhuman. There are two types of asocial predator:

o Asocial resource predators are scavengers. You can sometimes give up a material thing and be safe.

o Asocial process predators want to do things; they will want you in a private place under their control. Never be seduced by charm or promises and do whatever you must to avoid being lured to a secondary location.

Suggested Practice

 Think Like Professor Moriarty: figure out how to acquire something you want without getting caught. What are the steps? What are the dangers? Forget ethical considerations.

What would you do to survive if you were suddenly evicted and had no friends or family to lean on? If after a few weeks on the street you had become invisible and begging didn't supply enough money for food or medicine? What if there were a real possibility you might lose a child to hunger or illness? What are your options? How do they play out?

There are endless versions of this thought experiment meant to create a deeper understanding of alternate states of mind and the behavior that might follow. Here's another…

Look at your home. Walk around the outside. Imagine you've been locked out and your child is in danger. How would you get inside?

CHAPTER 4

Prey or Privilege

We are what we think; all that we are arises with our thoughts, with our thoughts we make the world.
—Buddha

To be a predator is to hunt people for play or personal gain. To be prey is to lack choices and privileges. Let's assume it's best to have all the options of the predator but the intention to use those privileges wisely and generously.

Mind-Setting Part 2

We don't see things as they are, but as we are.
—Anais Nin

We might describe mindset loosely as a collection of beliefs and attitudes shaped by our experiences, shifting fluidly with emotion and circumstance, and continually influencing how we perceive ourselves and others. The mindset we occupy at any given moment can have a significant impact on the experience of that moment and on outcome, because mindset is not just a lens though which we see and process the world; it is also a lens through which the world sees and processes us.

In protective offense, mindset is central. Our mindset dictates the tools at our disposal at any given moment. With a subservient mindset, we may wait for a situation to change on its own; in a proactive mindset, we put ourselves in a mental position to lead and problem-solve. There's a qualitative difference that moves the world around us.

Like a house with many windows, we may shift mindsets depending on where we are and who we are with. We are in a different mindset when we visit our parents than we are when we go to work. We choose different mindsets for different purposes, but emotion makes things slippery, and most often mindset chooses us.

Clearly, we are not responsible for everything negative that happens to us, but what if there were a confluence of personal characteristics that could make us a potential target of crime? What if individually these characteristics wouldn't cause much trouble, but if they flocked together they could attract predators like blood in the water?

In the last chapter, we studied a combination of attributes common to criminals and predators. In this chapter, let's turn that x-ray vision on ourselves. Our ability to witness our own mindset is a main aspect that separates humans from other animals; we have an experience, we have sensory and emotional data related to the experience, then we have thoughts about that data—thoughts about how we think, feel, and respond to a particular experience. Sometimes those cognitive processes happen nearly simultaneously, and our thoughts about how we are thinking can redirect our behavior. That ability to self-monitor, to step outside and watch our own brains at work, is a key factor in the human story.

Start listening to your own brain whizzing away, watch it at work, train it to be honest with you. Don't get angry or frustrated when it doesn't work the way you want it to; treat it like a child or a puppy and train it with curiosity and encouragement. We never received a manual for this apparatus, so give yourself space to explore. Our best work is often done under the care of the teacher who liked us most, who stimulated us into our deepest creativity and made us feel excited about what we could accomplish.

The ability to analyze and adjust our behavior is a superpower that, aside from helping us avoid trouble, can also enable us to live a more effective and satisfying life. This is not changing to suit others, but the opportunity to consider our contribution to any interaction and to choose a particular trajectory. What we say and do influences everyone around us and could have a significant effect on the reactions of a violent personality. Everyone has an opinion about what the other guy should do—about how to fix rapists or the criminal justice system—but how many of us spend time fixing our own behavior? We are all connected.

Becoming an anti-target is a process of shoring up chinks in your armor. There is no such thing as a house that is impervious. Even an underground bomb shelter can be found and breached by professionals. We want to become (or for our students to become) invisible, or at least to make it more difficult and less fun to perpetrate a crime against us. Each step is another hoop for a criminal to jump through, intended to discourage him from focusing on us as a target.

Following is a list of habits or traits to help remove us from the criminal radar. We must examine ourselves first before we can pass these skill sets on to our friends, children, and students.

Twelve Traits of Protective Offense

1. **Personal Responsibility**

    I am responsible for my own protection. I don't expect others—the police, firefighters, lawyers, even doctors—to be my or my family's sole, or even primary, protectors.

    I accept responsibility for my part in any interaction and try not to blame others for things within my control.

    Civilization supplies us with HGTV and heated car seats, but the unfortunate side effect is that we become comfortably numb and abandon responsibility for our safety to others. We allow doctors, lawyers, and police to guide us and manage important aspects of our lives, and we hope they have the best intentions. But everything works better if we do our part.

    We are often the cause of our own woes. This is not a popular way of looking at things, but it is an effective one. We cannot change other people's behavior, but we can identify our own glitches, recalibrate, and avoid quite a bit of mayhem.

2. **Acceptance of Risk**
   I accept that predators are part of life and that I cannot change this fact. When I spend time asking why this must be, I miss the chance to ask more insightful questions.
   I accept the conveniences and inconveniences that come with living in society. Though I have the freedom to do, wear, or say what I want, I calculate the risk of attracting unwanted or unexpected consequences and plan ahead.
   I accept that some rules and standards are unfair, but reasonable allowances must be made for the existence of other people. And unfairness is part of what makes women unsafe and must always be accounted for.

3. **Health Before Vice or Vanity**
   I know that studying self-defense without making the best choices I can about my general health is like planning to protect myself from an attacker while standing on quicksand. I prioritize personal health, strength, flexibility, and balance training as much as possible because muscle mass and mobility increase my resilience to danger.[10] I know that even from a distance my posture loudly signals my ability or inability to protect myself, so when I exercise I always emphasize correct posture.
   I try to wear shoes and clothing that make it easy for me to move and breathe. I don't want to be at the mercy of my clothing in an emergency. I am aware that heels are damaging to my feet and posture and know that they sound like a dinner bell to predators, so I carry them with me and wear good shoes for moving.
   I know breathing is central to health so I try not to wear anything that constricts my waist or diaphragm that forces me to raise my shoulders when I breathe and may encourage my nervous system to be in fight or flight.
   I try to be aware of how things I consume affect me physically and mentally. I know certain drugs, processed foods, alcohol, artificial sweeteners, sugar, and even caffeine can cause allergies, sleep disorders, auto-immune responses, and mood swings.

---

10 Justin C. Brown, Michael O. Harhay, and Meera N. Harhay, "Sarcopenia and Mortality among a Population-Based Sample of Community-Dwelling Older Adults," *Journal of Cachexia, Sarcopenia and Muscle* 7, no. 3 (June 2016): 290–98, https://doi.org/10.1002/jcsm.12073.

There seemed to be a limitless number of objects in the world that had no practical use but that people wanted to preserve… There were a number of impractical shoes, stilettos mostly, beautiful and strange.
      —*Station Eleven*, Emily St. John Mandel

4. **Preparation**

   I believe preparation helps me avoid rushing and gives me an edge over chaos. This extra step keeps me from get lost, forgetting important things, or becoming dangerously distracted. I carve out five minutes or so each morning or evening to create a basic mental or written map of my day. I prepare with extra care when traveling or doing anything new or unusual. I refuse to be thought of as flaky or unreliable, so I leave extra time for traffic and other unavoidable inconveniences. Knowing change is the only constant, I remain flexible and ready to recalculate.

Doing something quickly prevents it from being done well.
      —Old Chinese adage

I do one thing… I do it well… then I move on.
      —Charles Emerson Winchester III, from *M.A.S.H.*

5. **Situational Awareness, Active Listening, Intuition**

   Predators seek out distracted people, so I take in my surroundings and try not to zone out randomly; I gather information and heed the subtle voices in my head. I keep my eyes up and my mind present. I seek first to understand and avoid beginning sentences with the words, "No, but…" I never want to assume I have all the information, or make decisions based on incomplete or faulty information. My intuition is formed by a combination of life experience, instinct, and sensory input, all combined into a wonderous alert system. It has served me well many times and I always listen when it calls.

6. **Verbal Communication: Voice Control and Modulation**

   I try to speak lower and slower because I know high-pitched, quick speech sends a message of nervous distraction, desperation, or validation seeking. I try to be aware of the signals I give off and modulate my speech for effective and self-aware communication.

7. **Nonverbal Communication**
   I am aware of how my facial expressions and body language affect interactions with others. I know wearing my distaste face at the wrong time may adversely affect my goals and even create conflict. I know that lip-pursing is a sign I'm hyper-focused, and wincing excessively while searching for something in my bag is a request for validation. I know my posture expresses how able I am to protect myself and others. I am aware that these signals may invite or deter predators.

   Can't read my, can't read my,
   no he can't read my poker face...
       —Lady Gaga, "Poker Face"

8. **Optimal Decision-Making Using Emotion, Logic, Experience, and Intuition in Symphony.**
   I know how to listen to my emotions without being controlled by personal drama. I am aware that leaning too hard on logic may cause me to miss emotional cues and misunderstand motivations. Experience guides and educates me. Intuition spins a web between all my resources. My life is mostly a product of my decisions, and I use all my skills to inform and guide me.

   > Intuition is not infallible. A child who associates a bearded doctor with pain may harbor an unfair bias against men with beards. The sense of foreboding you feel around your BFF's new boyfriend may or may not be justified. Listen first, then interrogate your intuition and decide when it warrants a closer look.

9. **Set Boundaries: Be Respectful and Empathetic but Assertive**
   I know niceness may be seen as indecision or even subservience and may cause asocial people to disregard or manipulate me. I am clear with myself first before I set and enforce my boundaries. I consider myself fair-minded, respectful, and decent but assertive.

10. **Self-Awareness and Auto-Correction**
    I try to be aware of the inner workings of my mind and seek to adjust repetitive problematic behavior. Statistics say people I know or with whom I have regular contact are more likely to

cause me harm, and that if they know my weaknesses, schedule, or behavioral patterns they may be capable of exploiting those things. Working on myself keeps my mind supple and helps me avoid traps caused by lazy thinking.

Master your mind to master any conflict.
—Takuan Sōhō, *The Unfettered Mind*

11. **Seek Knowledge**
I like to keep my mind strong and flexible. Whenever I feel myself stagnating, I know it's time to read or learn something new. Staying creative and open to new ways of thinking helps me find solutions and experience potentially stressful interactions as opportunities to learn or reevaluate what I think I already know.

The great secret to safety and dynamic living is not in my body but my mind. The people who survive and thrive are not bigger and stronger, they are creative and resilient, always gathering information and recalibrating.

12. **Inner Peace: Rest, De-Stress, and Seek Wonder**
I prioritize recovery because stress is at the root of some of the most insidious outcomes and blocks intuitive signals with harmful static. Stress causes me to yell at someone who just happens to be having the worst day of their life, which causes them to make it the worst day of mine. It causes a plethora of prey signals that can be picked up on and exploited by criminals and keeps me stuck in repetitive problematic behaviors; it prevents me from planning, speaking slowly and clearly, and exhibiting my best behavior in general.

Much of the trouble in my life occurs when I am in a rush, unprepared, tired, angry, distracted, or overwhelmed. I seek moments of joy and wonder, whether it's walking in nature, making art, or laughing with a friend. I know that when I don't stop to breathe and feel joy, life feels small and overcrowded and I miss important signals and make unfortunate decisions.

Ideally, I try to get to the root causes of stress in my life because I know that trying to mitigate stress while the stressor persists is like trying to fix an overflowing sink by throwing buckets of water out the window.

Recap

- Mindset drives our responses but also dictates the way the world responds to us.
    - Train your brain to be honest with you. Being able to analyze and adjust your behavior is a superpower.
    - Staying off the criminal radar is a process. Even an underground bomb shelter can be breached by professionals. Make it more difficult to get to you and your family.
- Use the Twelve Traits of Protective Offense to keep you off the criminal radar.

Suggested Practices

Look at yourself from a criminal's viewpoint. How easy a target are you mentally, emotionally, physically? Take a good look at the way you move through the world. Find your blind spots, pick one, make a plan, and go to work. Tiny changes accumulate; they're also easier to make than large ones. This may all seem peripheral. It's not. We often think of physical strength as the gateway to safety, but overall health, focus, and mental fortitude work better to keep you off the criminal radar and make you safer and more effective in so many ways.

Pick one of the Twelve Traits of Protective Offense. Here are some ideas:

 Cultivate Trait 3: Health Before Vice or Vanity by looking for any opportunity to move and improve functional strength and posture. Don't wait for the gym; the world is your playground. Walk instead of taking the car or bus. Rollerblade, ride your bike, or scooter like a kid. Avoid elevators and climb stairs at every opportunity. Help a friend move into their new house. Carry your neighbor's groceries up six flights. Don't stagnate in a chair (one of our worst inventions—we evolved to sit cross-legged or to squat), get up every hour to move, or do five minutes of chair yoga (since you're in the chair anyway). A few more minutes per hour of movement can quickly add up to an hour a day of oxygen in your blood, better sleep, and health.

These practices also positively affect Trait 7: Nonverbal Communication. Posture collapses as we age. Even from a distance, vitality and posture telegraph strength, agility, speed, and health, all things predators check for in their victims.

> Look into my favorite strength workouts, Functional Range Conditioning (FRC) and KinStretch (the "k" is for "kinetic")—the internal martial arts answer to hardcore strength training. Difficult to explain (even more difficult to do), think yoga and Pilates on steroids. Works as physical therapy for many injuries and chronic conditions or to break plateaus and leap ahead as a professional athlete. Takes heart and tons of focus, but the benefits are mind-blowing. Albis Suarez has been my trainer for many years. Find him at movebetterwithalbis.com.

 Cultivate Trait 4: Preparation by carving out five minutes each evening to plan the next day and five minutes in the morning to modify it. Leave room for change—it's the only constant. Do it in your head, on paper, on your phone. If you're doing something different than usual—like taking a long trip—leave time for research or to consider the most likely snafus. Keep a map in the car in case your phone dies or lacks connection. Bring extra food and water. A first-aid kit is never a bad idea (more in chapter 11). Be reasonable about what you can get done in a day; rushing and lack of planning are an emergency's best friends.

 Cultivate Trait 6: Verbal Communication—Voice Control and Modulation

- **Record your voice relaxed and under duress** It's invaluable to know how you sound under stress (find that video of yourself at the family reunion). What we see in the mirror is the reverse of what others see. Voices are different too.
- **Try a voice stress test.** See if you can control your voice after vigorous exercise. Go for lower and slower. Try to keep your voice calm even when you're out of breath.

- **Breath control** is a powerful way to change the register of your voice and help you control your reaction to cortisol and adrenaline. Breathwork has many benefits. More on breathing in chapter 10.

Cultivate Trait 7: Consider Observing Your Emotional Expressions in the Mirror or on Video.

This can be difficult to do spontaneously but it's worth trying. It can be helpful to know if you look angry when you're tired, or disgusted when you mean to look confused. Misunderstandings cause us a lot of trouble.

Cultivate Trait 10: Self-Awareness and Auto-Corrective Behavior

Observe your own behavior to find and fix behavioral glitches. What are your go-to reactions? Patterns indicate habits. By practicing self-observation, we learn to spot problematic behaviors in others. A good place to try this is while driving or interacting with your kids or pets. How quickly do you get angry when someone cuts you off or steals your parking space? Or when your child disregards you loudly in public?

- Does the feeling last or come and go quickly?
- Do you take things personally?
- Do you feel like there has to be payback?
- Do you let people tell their story, or do you talk over them and insist on your version of events?
- Do you let people get away with everything and fail to be assertive when it's called for?
- Do you generally react aggressively or timidly? Or do you respond with calm reason?

Cultivate Trait 12: Inner Peace: Rest, Release Stress, and Seek Wonder

Acquire some stress-releasing skills. Schedule a few moments of reprieve, and make a contract with yourself that becomes habit.

- **Make an agreement with a friend to check in** and vent or just listen once a week.
- Schedule fifteen minutes to unabashedly **play with your dog or kids.**

- Try a **morning walk in nature** first thing, standing with your face toward the sky, feeling good in your skin, even if you just pretend. Being sad under a tree is better than being sad under artificial lighting.
- **Learn how to meditate.** You don't have to empty your mind or even sit completely still. This misinformation keeps us from trying. You're allowed to scratch your nose. Find a reputable practitioner live or online. You'll find meditation tips in chapter 10.
- **Think about your stress differently.** If you haven't already, watch Kelly McGonigal's TED Talk "How to Make Stress Your Friend."

PART 3

THE SELF-DEFENSE CONTINUUM

CHAPTER 5

The Self-Defense Continuum—Overview

When my son was born, his ears were translucent. He was so tiny, so horrifyingly fragile, and I was overwhelmed with a desperate need to protect him from everything. Yet, when I began to run scenarios in my mind detailing how a crime against me might play out—how I would protect my infant in an encounter with a desperate, drug-addled troublemaker—what I came up with was utterly inadequate: talk my way out of it, run while trying to protect my baby's delicate neck from my jarring movements. Perhaps. But how could I possibly fight while wearing him on the front of my body as a shield?

My mind worked furiously in those days, searching for a formula that alleviated my hypervigilant mommy brain. I went back to the proverbial drawing board, beginning not with fighting or martial arts, but with conflict and crime and how I would have to circumvent it as a mother. It helped to break moments into more accessible pieces—to demystify crime by seeing it as a process rather than a sudden occurrence.

I looked at a well-known model used by law-enforcement called the Crime Triangle. This model names the points of a triangle—motive, means, and opportunity—and posits that if any side of the triangle is removed, a crime cannot occur. The Triangle is often used retrospectively to ascertain if a suspect could have perpetrated a crime. It is sometimes also used to illustrate how we have the most control over removing opportunity. While this is a great model in its simplicity, I was in search of something that provided more insight.

I began seeking out martial artists who were also looking to examine blind spots. It was during this time that I connected with Marc MacYoung and Erik Kondo. Erik Kondo is a high-level jujitsu stylist and conflict analyst who, because he spends his waking hours in a wheelchair, has an unusually enlightened insight into self-defense. Erik created the Five Ds of Self-Defense, five steps for avoiding and escaping crime that have been used by law enforcement for years. The Five Ds are Decide, Deter, Disrupt, Disengage, and Debrief. Marc MacYoung is a long-time bouncer, conflict analyst, expert witness in self-defense cases and the author of many excellent books on violence. Marc created the Five Stages of Violent Crime, an internationally recognized system to identify the development specifically of violent crime. The Five Stages are Intent, Interview, Positioning, Attack, and Reaction.

In a turn of serendipity, I saw that Marc and Erik had each come up with mnemonic devices that completed each other. Erik's Five Ds and Marc's Five Stages formed the Self-Defense Continuum (SDC), which I used as a model to articulate the seemingly random, surprising, often incomprehensible process of crime, and to highlight the most urgent control points where a potential target might affect the outcome of a crime. Like the Five Stages of Grief (denial, anger, bargaining, depression, and acceptance) the SDC helps us find patterns and interject solutions.

On his encyclopedic website about violence, NoNonsenseSelfDefense.com (also NNSD.com), Marc writes that, perhaps counterintuitively, it may seem that the odds are in favor of the criminal, but instead the criminal's goals can make him predictable. He uses an analogy of driving to a destination; when you start out, there are many roads you can take to get there, but the closer you get, the fewer the options that will take you where you want to go. Marc says, "The closer to the commission of the crime, the more predictable the criminal becomes… it is that predictability that you can turn against him to ensure your safety."

Chapter 5: The Self-Defense Continuum—Overview

This introductory chapter serves as an outline for the next five lessons that expound on each section of the continuum. Here's how it works:

THE SELF~DEFENSE CONTINUUM					
Erik Kondo's 5 Ds of Self-Defense describe the offensive steps you take to avoid or survive violence and other crimes					
DECIDE	DETER	DISRUPT	DISENGAGE		DEBRIEF
Before		During			After
INTENT	INTERVIEW	POSITIONING		ATTACK	REACTION
Marc MacYoung's 5 Stages of Violent Crime describe the steps a predator takes to commit violence and other crimes					

In the graphic (above), between the Five Ds of Self-Defense and the Five Stages of Violent Crime, you see the words Before, During, and After. Each phase of the criminal process tends to occur at a point along the continuum. Intent generally occurs before a criminal carries out an attack; if you miss intent, the interview might occur around the same time or just after. Positioning and attack make up the during stage because this is the most common chronology. Reaction concludes the timeline in the after stage.

I explain this framework in a moment, but first I want to point out that this is not by any means the only way crimes happen, and to fixate on the chronology is to risk creating a faulty mental model and missing the available signs. We are working within a model, and all models are necessarily artificial and inherently imperfect. The stages don't always happen cleanly and separately; sometimes they overlap or happen simultaneously—human behavior is not a mathematical formula. So, if you always look for intent to happen first, you may miss it. The stages of the SDC are for reference and comprehension. They are not static. It is entirely possible for intent to occur in the moment because a desperate criminal finds you alone in a dark parking lot searching in your purse for your keys. In this case, positioning came first, then intent, then interview. This is often the case in crimes of opportunity. The way to avoid these types of crimes is by never presenting yourself as an opportunity too good to pass up. This happens in the decide stage of the SDC, which we will cover in the next chapter. We are using the Self-Defense Continuum to slow down the process of crime and break it into stages while also being purposely vague about what the intended crime might be to make the model more applicable to multiple situations.

Let's break it down. Though Erik's Five Ds are at the top of the SDC graphic to highlight our control points, I'm going to start with Marc's Five Stages to make it clear what we're up against.

Why does a criminal need to take any particular steps? Because if he picks the wrong person and you happen to be a police officer or a citizen with a weapon, he may be hurt or caught. So, one of the first things he must do is observe you.

Crime often begins with intent, which is different than motive in that it is a completed decision. You can be motivated to do something but not ready or prepared to do it. Many of us are motivated to lose weight or to change jobs, but that doesn't mean it will happen. Intent implies readiness and commitment, sometimes desperation. A crime begins when a criminal decides they need something badly enough that they are willing to shoulder a certain amount of risk to acquire it.

The interview stage is the moment in which a criminal gathers information about you and evaluates your suitability as a victim. A criminal may covet you from afar rather than talk to you. He may gather information by observation or through your friends and acquaintances. He might hide behind the internet and pose as someone younger, older, of a different gender, or of a certain political or religious affiliation. By posing as someone who has something in common with the target, or as someone nonthreatening, a criminal gains access to private lives and the confidence of vulnerable strangers. Questions might begin with the innocuous and become gradually more specific and personal. We are all vulnerable at points in our lives, and when we crave connection we ignore our intuition and become easier targets (more on this next chapter in the section called "Wanting").

> A few years ago, Erik Kondo began a group for physically disabled women preyed upon by fetishists. These men masqueraded as other disabled women—friendships formed, intimate secrets were shared. Reading the communications, Kondo found incongruities, odd lines of questioning—clues to deception that we are more likely to catch and act on with a little awareness of how they work.

Chapter 5: The Self-Defense Continuum—Overview

Positioning is often the next stage of a crime. Once a criminal has interviewed you and decided you are a suitable target, they need to get to a place (or move you to a place) where they can successfully control you. This includes getting you into an emotional position to accept the abuse (see "Devious Tactics" in the next chapter). A criminal will bring to bear any tool or ploy that will allow them to get close to you: charm, force, and everything in between. Sometimes the criminal will spend most of their time in the intent and interview stages to determine whether you are likely to fight back. In a purse-snatching, the positioning stage can be very short.

However, as discussed earlier in the case of a positioning-based attack, like a crime of opportunity, the intent to find the right moment to score was inherent and positioning might be the first stage of the crime you detect.

Once a criminal sets his intent, interviews you, and gets into position, he will progress to the attack stage, which can mean anything from a simple robbery to something worse. This is where a criminal corners or puts hands on you and your options diminish drastically.

You begin to see why using the continuum and responding early is at least as helpful as leaning on currently accepted forms of physical self-defense as a final response to a potentially avoidable catastrophe.

The criminal reaction occurs after the attack when emotions are high. Criminals don't always plan past the main event, and plans don't always go as expected. An assailant may have the intention of killing you but guilt may change the plan. Or it can go the other way. He may have planned to escape quickly, but now you're mouthing off, so his finger somehow finds its way to the trigger. Attackers are often people known to us, and high emotion can act like gasoline on a fire—adrenaline and cortisol are powerful drugs. The reaction stage can be crucial since a criminal's erratic and unpredictable behavior—and yours—can have lasting repercussions. More than one assailant means more emotions. If your assailants disagree about what to do, it can create an aftershock to rival the original attack. If you get away, you may still be so panicked that you run into an oncoming truck. It isn't over until it's over. Even weeks, months, or years later, PTSD can have a lasting impact.

Erik Kondo's Five Ds of Self-Defense give you the action steps to counter a criminal's progress against you.

The first D is decide. The decide stage of the continuum is rather nebulous and includes all manner of education and preparation. You decided to read this book, which is full of decide skills, among them becoming more self-aware, learning about predators, becoming an active observer, and improving your decision-making abilities. With regards to the SDC, we will be discussing decide as it relates to its counterpart, intent.

When we combine the top and bottom boxes at each stage of the SDC, we get what we must do to counter a criminal's plans. In this first stage, we could call the combination Decide to Recognize Intent. This is the title of chapter 6, where we will decide to learn about the signs of intent so we can halt the progress of crime.

The next stage of The Five D's is deter, which is what we want to do when a criminal tries to interview us for the role of victim. So chapter 7, called Deter the Interview, is where we cover nuanced skills like de-escalation and boundary-setting.

Chapter 8 will be called Disrupt Positioning. Here we will consider skills to keep a criminal from moving into a position where he can successfully subdue or attack you.

Chapter 9, Disengage the Attack, is the stage that requires you to get physical as your last and best chance of escape or survival.

Chapter 10, Debrief After the Reaction, is where we mitigate any further physical or emotional damage, learn from our mistakes, and heal intelligently. It is a part of the timeline that's rarely discussed. Here we will cover short- and long-term debriefing strategies for working through the aftermath of a violent encounter.

The process of crime or event prediction is very much about seeing and understanding more than we thought was there. If you have ever traveled to a foreign country and didn't speak the language, you might remember consciously or unconsciously shutting out what you didn't understand to diminish stress. The language and behavior of devious people is in many cases foreign to us, so we miss it, shut it out, or translate it improperly. The less familiar a situation, the more sudden and jarring it feels. When we are blind to a process, we are unable to

Chapter 5: The Self-Defense Continuum—Overview

comprehend it, let alone affect it, and the way we process information expands or contracts our sense of time.

The OODA Loop—sometimes fondly referred to as OODA Loops—is not a sugary kid's cereal but a model developed by military strategist and Air Force colonel John Boyd. OODA stands for Observe, Orient, Decide, Act and describes the process the brain undergoes when confronted with unfamiliar information. The OODA mental model has been applied to many decision-making processes (most notably law enforcement, litigation, and business) and provides an explanation for the freeze response—that deer-in-headlights moment we have when the radically unexpected occurs. When we can't properly orient and observe, the brain loops, searching for an acceptable next move, and is unable to decide or act.

The SDC helps us make sense of self-defense. It helps us move more quickly through the OODA process by demystifying the steps to a crime, allowing us to spot incidents sooner, and affording more time for crucial calculations.

> *When you react, the event controls you.*
> *When you respond, you're in control.*
> —Dr. George Thompson, *Verbal Judo: The Gentle Art of Persuasion*

Recap

- The Self-Defense Continuum (SDC) is a model that combines Marc MacYoung's Five Stages of Violent Crime: Intent, Interview, Positioning, Attack, and Reaction; and Erik Kondo's Five Ds of Self-Defense: Decide, Deter, Disrupt, Disengage, and Debrief.
- The SDC provides a framework for something normally viewed as incomprehensible. It artificially breaks the process of crime into stages while also being purposely vague to be more applicable to multiple situations.
- Criminals make decisions to avoid being hurt or caught, so they must first observe you. The process of crime or event prediction is very much about being aware and seeing more than we thought was there.

- John Boyd's OODA Loop describes the process the brain undergoes when confronted with unfamiliar information. The SDC helps us understand the inner workings of crime so we move more quickly through the OODA process, without losing life-saving seconds when it counts.

Suggested Practices

 Print the Self-Defense Continuum handout from ReimaginingWomensSelfDefense.com and put it somewhere useful. It is designed to be hung or folded into a bookmark.

 Set it and forget it. We spend a lot of time on autopilot. Stopping to consciously consider what we normally do by rote can bring our attention to blind spots and glitches in our habits and behaviors, especially if we have a habit of flying by the seat of our pants or running on fumes. Try setting random daily alarms on your phone, and when they go off take a moment to ask yourself three or more of the following questions:

- Am I in a familiar or unfamiliar place? Do I know where I'm going?
- How do I feel? Am I tired or hungry?
- Am I prepared for the day?
- Have I been paying attention or am I distracted? Am I in my phone or in the world?
- Am I in a rush?
- Am I alone or responsible for another?
- If driving, is my car inspected? Tires full of air? Gas tank at least half full? Am I overdue for an oil change?
- If walking, is my bag open? Hanging off my shoulder? Do I know where my wallet and keys are?
- What is my emotional state?
- How would I respond to something unexpected in this moment?
- Do I feel confident and able to handle annoying people or a sudden change of plans?
- Is my phone charged? Do I have anything at my immediate disposal that I could quickly use as a weapon if needed? (More on weapons later.)

CHAPTER 6

The Self-Defense Continuum, Stage 1— Decide to Recognize Intent

THE SELF~DEFENSE CONTINUUM					
Erik Kondo's 5 Ds of Self-Defense describe the offensive steps you take to avoid or survive violence and other crimes					
DECIDE	DETER	DISRUPT	DISENGAGE		DEBRIEF
Before		During			After
INTENT	INTERVIEW	POSITIONING	ATTACK		REACTION
Marc MacYoung's 5 Stages of Violent Crime describe the steps a predator takes to commit violence and other crimes					

SDC Stage 1: Decide/Intent

The fight is won or lost far away from witnesses—behind the lines, in the gym, and out there on the road, long before I dance under those lights.
—Muhammad Ali

We begin in the all-important before phase of the Self-Defense Continuum. Since emergencies don't tend to happen every day, before is where we spend most of our time. Once something goes wrong, we are in the during phase where we no longer have time to decide, prepare, make leisurely decisions, or comb our hair—because it's on fire. Before a robbery, we can choose which locks to buy and compare prices; during, we can only escape or fight. You are in the before phase now as you read this book. It is before until something goes wrong. Before is where most of the work gets done.

Preparation and information gathering are some of the most important steps you can take before a journey. When you plan to hike up a mountain, what you know and what you decide to carry with you make all the difference. There are infinite possibilities in the decide stage. You might decide to create a community of women in your neighborhood and plan to watch out for each other and stay informed about neighborhood activity; you might start a protective offense book club and choose books from the reading list to continue your learning and empower others; you might decide to make a checklist of ways to secure your home or create a comprehensive family first-aid kit and spend a few weekend hours on the project as per chapter 11. Decide includes anything you can do that improves your odds of avoiding or surviving a violent crime. This is the crux of the study of self-defense.

As per the SDC, however, we are going to Decide to Recognize Intent, which means focusing specifically on ways of recognizing the intent of another human to harm you or someone you care for.

> *The best defense against bullshit is vigilance.*
> *If you smell something, say something.*
> —Jon Stewart

In terms of the SDC, intent refers to a person's readiness to commit a crime. Intent is sometimes referred to as "motive," but I've also heard it called "desire." Without becoming bogged down in semantics, let's say desire and motive are precursors to intent, but that intent goes beyond. We all have good reasons to do lots of things we don't do. You could desire or be motivated to quit your job, but that doesn't mean you will. Intent is imminent.

Before you can thwart criminal intent you have to learn to recognize it, and the earlier you do so the better. Time equals options. When your intuition, informed by knowledge and experience, is doing its job, you won't even be sure danger was imminent. You will have responded by way of what *Gift of Fear* author Gavin de Becker calls the Messengers of Intuition: inarticulable doubt, nagging feelings, hesitation, suspicion, and true fear, among other signals. You will have changed your location or your behavior, ducked into a crowded well-lit store, decided not to have drinks with the guy you met at that thing, decided not to take the same route home you always take. You do these things not with a feeling of concern or inconvenience, but with an empowering sense of intuitive intelligence.

Things we have no experience with sometimes catch us off guard because they don't light up our intuition or sense of danger. Since you can only respond to what you know is problematic, knowledge of behaviors or dangers you want to avoid expands your intuition. It's like cooking with a slew of new ingredients.

Awareness Part 2: You See But You Do Not Observe

> *Unagi is a state of total awareness. Only by achieving true unagi can you be prepared for any danger that may befall you.*
> —Ross, from *Friends*

The professor at the head of the class replies to an incorrect student assessment, "The gentleman has ears and he hears not, eyes and he sees not." If this sounds like Sherlock Holmes, it's because professor of surgery, Dr. Joseph Bell, was Arther Connan Doyle's inspiration for his famous fictional character. It was Bell who reportedly said, "Glance at a man and you find his nationality written on his face, his means of livelihood on his hands, and the rest of his story in his gait, mannerisms, watch-chain ornaments, and the lint adhering to his clothes."

Beyond relaxed awareness, we could add focused attention or observation, a deeper, more nuanced examination that can be practiced. In the martial arts, the military, and some dangerous jobs you will hear about situational awareness. The term originated in the military and refers to the ability to perceive multiple elements in a dynamic environment, comprehend how they interact, and project a general outcome. It is a highly nuanced and sought-after ability that involves actively observing all elements of your immediate surroundings, including people and behavior, objects and obstacles, and environmental conditions like weather or pollution levels. Inadequate situational awareness is considered a primary factor in accidents stemming from human error.

Dr. Mica Endsley, one of the foremost authorities on the subject,[11] breaks situational awareness into the following steps:

1. **Perception:** be aware of the relevant elements in the environment. Observe and gather both sensory and external information about the status and dynamics of an environment and its respective components: people, objects, and events.
2. **Comprehension:** understand the meaning of those elements and their relationship. Organize information using pattern recognition, interpretation, and evaluation to form a mental model of the situation.
3. **Projection:** anticipate future status or events based on current understanding.

Dr. Endsley's detailed step-by-step clarification illustrates that situational awareness requires a deeper, more nuanced form of observation and information gathering than you would normally use. Clearly, this is a scientific model, not one meant to be followed word-for-word on a daily basis. Though detailed, if I had asked you to explain the steps to a heightened form of awareness, you might have come up with some of these same concepts.

Leonardo da Vinci attributed his accomplishments to what he called saper vedere or knowing how to see. He wrote that discovery was 90 percent observation. Isaac Newton said, "If I have ever made valuable discoveries, it has been owing more to patient attention than to any other talent."

---

11 Micah Endsley, "Toward a Theory of Situation Awareness in Dynamic Systems," *Human Factors* 37, no. 1 (March 1995): 32–64, https://doi.org/10.1518/001872095779049543.

Chapter 6: The Self-Defense Continuum, Stage 1

With all the external noise of daily life, how do we learn to cultivate focused observation? Luckily, it seems that neural pathways can be rewired and strengthened at any age. Multiple studies published by the *Journal of Vision* confirm that we can significantly increase attention by engaging in challenging visual attention tasks. Though observation involves more than just our eyes, sighted humans lean most heavily on sight for information gathering. Image processing uses 25 percent of our brain and more than 65 percent of our brain pathways. Samuel Renshaw, an American psychologist whose research on vision was instrumental in helping the armed forces quickly recognize enemy aircraft in World War II, said proper seeing is a skill like playing the piano—the eyes can be trained just as fingers can.

A visual model for stronger observation skills can be found in Amy Herman's Art of Perception program, which she teaches to the FBI, Fortune 500 companies, and the Department of Defense, among many others. The core of her program center around "the four A's"—how to assess, analyze, articulate, and adapt. She begins by helping students study the mechanics of sight and issues with perceptual filters and various types of cognitive biases. Assessment continues with what she calls "an orderly process for efficient, objective surveillance." The program continues with analysis—how to prioritize, recognize patterns, and differentiate between perception and inference. Articulation follows so students can pass their discoveries and help others see as well (an excellent skill for communicating with police or lawyers after an incident involving violence for the purpose of self-defense). Herman urges students to be specific, to use objective rather than subjective terms. She tells students to use descriptive adjectives to describe what they see rather than emotional interpretations; i.e., the subject of the painting is looking away with a turned-down mouth, rather than that the subject of the painting is sad, bashful, embarrassed, or shameful—all interpretations different people might have of the same expression. Finally, Herman teaches students to adapt their behavior based on the first three elements.

Herman cites numerous examples of acts of focused observation leading to major breakthroughs. In one instance, she tells the story of a hotel cleaner who noticed an empty room where a young girl sat, ill-dressed for the cold weather, without luggage and refusing to make eye contact. The observant cleaner reported what she saw and helped authorities reveal an international sex trafficking ring.

Herman calls on exercises in radical engagement (a term coined by writer Russell Carmony), including the intensive study of visual art, as a quantifiable way to test and improve observation. Students spend up to a few hours with a single piece of art, cataloging its elements and asking pointed questions like: What is going on in the painting? What relationships do you see between people and objects? What questions does the art elicit? She cites multiple studies on what humans fail to see right in front of them, how various cognitive biases work, and how we can disarm them. She encourages us her students and readers to ask more questions: What am I tuning out? What might I be taking for granted? What would someone else coming into my world not know? And the very important, What do I need to know?

Near the end of the book, Herman writes, "When you tap into your visual intelligence, you are transformed into a super sleuth, a case-cracker, and a guardian angel all in one. You feel like you've uncovered a secret world that's been right there all along." Best-selling author Dr. Wayne W. Dyer says, "Change the way you look at things and the things you look at change."

As a way to avoid danger, awareness and observation are crucial to safe and intelligent living. This book touches on many elements of protective offense but most skills herein require further study. You can read about Amy Herman's Art of Perception program in her book *Visual Intelligence*. There are multiple books on situational awareness, including Gary Quesenberry's excellent *Spotting Danger Before It Spots You*.

Nonverbal Deception

Many years ago, a man made a beeline toward my car, smiling. His trajectory was too direct and too fast, his smile too practiced. My three-year-old son was in the back seat. It was getting dark. The man held his hand out like he had a question, but I didn't see a question in his eyes. None of this was consciously thought out; I just responded to the discomfort I felt. I made my decision in maybe two seconds and rolled up my window while he closed distance. Part way, he called out something like, "Can I talk to you?" I pretended not to hear. I put the key in the ignition while he motioned for me to roll down the window and began to pull out slowly. He called out, but I was already too far to hear him. In my rearview mirror I saw his middle finger stab the air.

I love to help people. If you really need something, I'm your girl. But those were not the words or the body language of someone in need. I sensed an agenda—maybe not a dangerous agenda—but one I didn't feel I needed to be a part of. I'll never know what his intentions were, and that's okay with me. Good men who live in this world know that you don't rush up to a woman, especially one with a young child and at night. He may not have seen my son in the back seat, but I knew that something was off and that was good enough.

A lot goes on in a human interaction that isn't said with words. The study of nonverbal communication is the subject of constant conjecture. It is an imperfect science dependent on a multitude of changeable factors including the context of each interaction and also age, gender, and other variations in communicators. It is often stated that 80 percent of communication is nonverbal, but a deeper look shows this assertion dates back to a study done under specific circumstances and which involved a misapplication of the results.[12] More important than the numbers is the takeaway that when words don't seem properly matched to tone, expression, and posture, we lean more heavily on nonverbal data.

> *When there are inconsistencies between attitudes communicated verbally and posturally, the postural component should dominate in determining the total attitude that is inferred.*
> —Albert Mehrabian, behavioral scientist and author of *Nonverbal Communication*

---

[12] Paul Bell, "The Myths of Non-Verbal Communication: Revisiting Mehrabian and Its Misinterpretation in Corporate Training," *Australian Journal of Communication* 37, no. 3 (2010): 41–52.

According to a 2006 study, it appears that we are no more than 54-percent accurate at detecting lies.[13] This may be because laypeople have a truth bias and don't search for deception on a regular basis and professionals have a deception bias.

We are better at reading some cues than others and are far more accurate with people familiar to us than we are with strangers. Still, learning to understand nonverbal cues can help us recognize intent in someone wishing us harm if we use the knowledge holistically, in context, in the presence of other cues, and with special attention to incongruities between verbal and nonverbal cues.

What is the specific reason for an interaction (business or personal), the environment the interaction takes place in (crowded city, empty field), the roles of the people involved (husband and wife or teacher and student), the history between them (or lack thereof)? Someone who knows you well can touch your shoulder without it meaning anything discomfiting, not so for someone you've just met or a boss with whom you have a perfunctory relationship.

We don't have to study psychology, sociology, linguistics, haptics, mirroring, or proxemics to be decent people readers, but a more subtle understanding of these sciences can help us improve. Beware the urge to become a lie detection expert or to proclaim your knowledge of other people's mental and emotional states. You may be misleading yourself and making enemies in opposition to the goal of this book.

This short tutorial is meant to help you articulate some of the more important nonverbal behaviors that give you pause to further inform and train your intuition.

Eye contact and gaze behaviors are highly important forms of nonverbal communication. They can greatly affect an interaction and provide cues to what other people may be thinking or feeling. Eye contact communicates comfort, trust, or lack thereof, and provides cues to personality and confidence level. Too little eye contact or inability to maintain it may discredit what is being said or show lack of interest or disdain. Too much eye contact may appear suspicious—he could be showing attraction or aggression, trying to persuade or distract you.

---

13 Charles F. Bond and Bella M. DePaulo, "Accuracy of Deception Judgments," *Personality and Social Psychology Review* 10, no. 3 (August 2006): 214–34, https://doi.org/10.1207/s15327957pspr1003_2.

Chapter 6: The Self-Defense Continuum, Stage 1

Improper use of eye contact may cause discomfort, violate social rules, offend someone, or even insult them. Eye contact changes from culture to culture. In the West, looking a person in the eye demonstrates self-confidence and connection; in other places, a woman looking a man directly in the eye can be dangerous. Before traveling to an unfamiliar place, inquire about the rules of gesture and eye contact.

The assertion that blank or "empty" eyes are a sure sign of sociopathy is an oversimplification. Though faking emotional expression with the eyes is difficult, and a smile that doesn't involve puffed cheeks and eye crinkles might not be a true smile, expressions where the eyes don't participate should only be considered suspect in the company of other cues. Perhaps the eyes are incongruous with other body language cues or you sense a person is trying to mimic emotion with their eyes but their eyes are empty anyway. Blank eyes alone don't make a person dangerous, but it can be a piece of a greater story.

Facial expressions are central to communication; they enhance our words and elicit emotion. Empathy is the glue that binds us into communities. Your friend's sad expression causes *you* sadness. Often, changing your own expression can cause you to feel the emotion that goes with it. Expressions are driven by emotions, but the reverse can also be true.

Charles Darwin was the first to suggest that people express many emotions similarly, regardless of culture. Dr. Paul Ekman traveled far and wide to Japan, Chile, and even Papua New Guinea, among many other places, to confirm Darwin's hypothesis that expressions crossed cultures. Dr. Ekman categorized seven universal expressions that he even found in congenitally blind people who had never seen a human face. They are: happiness, surprise, anger, disgust, sadness, contempt, and fear.[14]

What I find most helpful is the simple act of articulating the differences among similar emotions like surprise and fear or anger, disgust, and contempt. Surprise and fear can be similar, but there are distinct differences. One difference is that surprised eyes are wide to take in as much information as possible. Fearful eyes try to hide the direction of their gaze so as not to telegraph important information. We also may sometimes confuse anger, disgust, and contempt. In both anger

---

[14] Paul Ekman Group, LLC, "Are There Universal Facial Expressions?," Paul Ekman Group, October 3, 2024, https://www.paulekman.com/resources/universal-facial-expressions/.

and disgust, the eyes are narrowed to try and hide any other emotional information that might leak, which is why those expressions also cause distrust in others. Contempt is similar to anger but asymmetrical in that one corner of the mouth is raised. Contempt often goes along with a sense of superiority, disregard, and disrespect, which makes it an expression to watch for.

In 1966, researchers distinguished micro-expressions from macro-expressions. Dr. Ekman is credited with expanding on the theory (the TV show *Lie to Me* is based on his work). Macro-expressions last longer than micro-expressions and match the general content and tone of the conversation or exchange. Micro-expressions only last around a fifteenth or twenty-fifth of a second and are accidental leaks that display concealed emotion or intention. This makes micro-expressions especially relevant for reading true intent when a person gives us pause. Micro-expressions are so fleeting they will mainly be caught subconsciously. When was the last time you had "a feeling," ignored it, and later thought, *I should have listened*? Micro-expressions can play a significant role in alerting our intuition when we can't quite explain why someone makes us uncomfortable.

Developed by anthropologist Edward T. Hall in the late 1950s, proxemics is the study of how people use space and how this affects social interaction. We use intimate space for close relationships, personal space for family and friends, social space for casual and professional relationships, and public space for strangers. When a stranger sits or stands too close—especially if there is space around him—how does it feel? Does it feel different when people face you directly or at an angle? I always find it odd when people in movies speak while facing each other directly. I find that casual conversations often occur at a forty-five-degree angle with intermittent eye contact. Find daily interactions and note how eye contact and proxemics affect how you feel about a person and an interaction. An understanding of basic proxemics is essential to proper boundary setting.

In 1977, Desmond Morris wrote *ManWatching, A Field Guide to Human Behavior*. In this definitive work, Morris includes facial expressions when he breaks body language into five categories: inborn, discovered, absorbed, trained, and mixed. He breaks gestures into thirteen

Chapter 6: The Self-Defense Continuum, Stage 1

more types and goes on to categorize a multitude of signs, signals, displays, nonverbal leakage, gaze behavior, and more. Without going into the vast complexities, what we can ultimately glean from Morris's work is that of all the body language categories, autonomic signals, which result from physiological changes beyond conscious control, are the most difficult to mask and therefore the most telling. Autonomic signals include signs of stress like fast breathing, sweating, excessive or arrested blinking, dry mouth, and pupil dilation. It is possible to change breathing or blinking rate temporarily, Morris notes, but the changes are difficult to maintain while also tending to other elements of deception. It is nearly impossible to consciously control sweating, and a dry mouth causes lip licking and other mouth movements that can be perceived and noted.

You are on vacation and your friend insists she is having a great time, yet she stops blinking when she says this, licks her lips repeatedly, and her shoulders are tensed. You sense something is up. You may find out later that she just received bad news and isn't quite ready to discuss it. Even without knowing the details, you put the signals together. Morris points to these contradictions between what is being said outright and autonomic body language as the best indicator of truth.

Anger signals can be important warnings, but not all anger looks the same. Sometimes anger is just overwrought frustration and isn't directed at anyone in particular, and other times it heralds the arrival of aggression. We are all familiar with the cartoon red face with steam bursting from the ears. According to Morris, facial pallor in anger is a more imminent sign of violence than redness. This is caused by the balancing actions of the sympathetic and parasympathetic areas of the nervous system. "If he is pale, he is more dangerous than if he has reddened," Morris explains, adding that pallor is part of the action system and indicates blood has been shunted to the arms and legs in preparation to fight or flee (note that Morris uses the word "pale," but darker skinned people may turn grayish or lack a healthy glow). Morris continues: "…if he is pale and approaching menacingly, he is likely to attack. But if he is bright red, it means he has already experienced the parasympathetic backlash and is no longer in the pure state of readiness…" The nervous system is adaptive, and so an angry red face is not to be trifled with either, but Morris calls the red face the result of an "impotent internal struggle that explodes in curses and roars and may seem alarming," but is often more a case of "bark being worse than bite."

Pupil dilation, another autonomic signal, is harder to notice but indicates a person excited into possible action. The pupils may widen to take in more information—is there someone around who might thwart their nefarious plan? Coupled with other anger signs, it can be an indicator of imminent action. That said, pupil dilation also happens when people are attracted to one another.

Other general anger signals include ones you're probably familiar with: nostril-flaring, eye-area tension, staring, sneering, frowning, foot stomping, fist clenching, chest puffing, teeth clenching, teeth licking with mouth open or closed, jaw thrusting, lip biting or clenching, and pounding on a surface with the hands or fist.

Some anger signals come in groups, like low frowning eyebrows with the head tilted downward, staring with lips pressed tightly, and nostrils flaring, or saber rattling, where someone deliberately messes with your stuff rather than messing with you, or invades your space to see if you will take the bait and escalate the game. Displays of anger may be deliberate attempts to get attention or a vent for built-up steam. An overt display of anger may suddenly turn aggressive even if it wasn't originally directed at you, or you could become collateral damage simply by being nearby. This is where active awareness plays a big role.

A threat display describes angry body language designed to intimidate an opponent into backing down. It says, "I'm bigger and badder, and you don't want to mess with me." Morris describes threat display gestures as attack actions that are cut off or checked before they make contact. Look for fists pounding the air, open hands slapping the air and stopping abruptly, wringing of an invisible rag or neck, clawed hands, fingers stabbing the air or cutting across the threatener's own throat.

Some threat displays occur more often between men—like chest puffing to appear larger and more intimidating. Threat displays against women are generally used for more covert and insidious purposes, such as to enforce subservience or to distract her into forgetting to protect herself. A person who has had an ugly experience with physical or emotional violence might freeze in the face of a threat display and be temporarily unable to act.

Finally, anger and threat displays can mask another devious intention: to provoke you into behavior that will in some way justify the abuse and subsequent escalation. Remember the earlier story about the ex-boyfriend who showed up at his ex-girlfriend's office while it was empty? Any form of intense anger whether repressed or overt should alert your protective instincts and cause you to de-escalate, move to safety, find help, or prepare for physical confrontation.

Anger isn't the only concerning sign. People making power plays or imposing dominance might sit or stand too close to you (remember the earlier discussion of proxemics) or touch you in casual yet vaguely inappropriate ways. They might "hood" by interlacing their arms behind their heads while talking to you to show you who's in charge. Both hands on a table with fingers spread wide is a territorial show of confidence and authority. Power plays are important signs that someone is trying to get you to make decisions in their best interest rather than your own.

> Don't take the bait. Anger is a "viral" emotion, and if you become caught up and mimic the same inflammatory behavior, you may inadvertently give an unstable person permission to escalate to violence. Engaging with him may play into Interview and Positioning. Attack comes next. Don't miss the signs of someone who is looking for "permission" to get physical.

Many expressions cross cultures, but nonverbal behaviors and gestures can be culture-specific in ways we haven't covered. For this reason, you might want to consult a native or a book on a specific culture when traveling to unfamiliar places.

A little knowledge is a dangerous thing.
—Alexander Pope

Lying is a specific form of deception. Where deception seeks to generally mislead or manipulate, lying involves deliberately providing false information. The science of lie detection is a topic of ongoing research and debate. Overconfidence is ill-advised. A little knowledge only helps if you respect it and use it wisely. While some nonverbal cues may indicate a lie, there is no reliable universal tell, and blogs that invite you to become a lie detection expert may be misleading or dangerous.

Research suggests that some nonverbal cues like fidgeting or avoiding eye contact may be associated with lying but may also signify general nervousness or discomfort. Though lying does use more energy and focus than telling the truth and sometimes causes obvious contradictions between verbal and physical cues (such as shaking the head no while saying yes, as seen in video footage of murderer Stephen McDaniel), it is important to approach lie detection with caution. Catching someone in a lie and calling them out on it may cause a backlash regardless of who is right.

Unfortunately, some sociopaths and psychopaths lack function in areas of the brain that differentiate between lies and truth and therefore don't display as many tells.[15] In this case, you will have to rely on multiple methods to recognize lying or intent.

Experts like Joe Navarro, a career FBI agent and author of *What Every Body Is Saying*, and Desmond Morris cite excessive face touching as a potential sign of lying or at least of stress. This includes gestures like partial mouth covering as a subconscious attempt to keep a lie from exiting the mouth. Eye blocking shields the brain from "seeing" the truth and communicates disdain. Nose touching, scratching, or rubbing may occur because the hand, on its way to cover the mouth, is caught and deflected to the nose. This may also occur due to the presence of erectile tissue in the anterior of the nose (responsible for congestion and decongestion) that is stimulated by the extra blood flow brought on by excitement (use that on trivia night!). You might see chin stroking or cheek rubbing, earlobe pulling, hair grooming, and eyebrow scratching or pinching (look for the eyebrow pinching scene in *Miracle on 34th Street*). Rubbing the forehead is often a signal someone is struggling with something. Remember that people also touch their faces when they have allergies or are tired, so it is by awareness of multiple signals in context that we eke out the truth.

---

15 R. J. R. Blair, "Applying a Cognitive Neuroscience Perspective to the Disorder of Psychopathy," *Biological Psychiatry* 57, no. 11 (2005): 119–26.

Chapter 6: The Self-Defense Continuum, Stage 1

Navarro cites signs of emotional discomfort or fear in self-pacifying behaviors like neck touching or stroking or fingers covering the suprasternal notch. You might see something he calls leg grooming where the legs are repeatedly rubbed or massaged. When a person is stressed or trying to self-empower, you might see the arms cross. Yawning is way of taking a deep breath and also causes the salivary glands to wet a dry mouth. Crossing the arms and rubbing from the shoulders down as if cold is another common pacifying behavior. Locking the feet around the legs of a chair is a minor sign of freeze and signifies anxiety or concern.

Other behaviors include self-ventilation due to the autonomic nervous system cooling the body with sweat. In this case, you would notice a shirt-flapping or hair-tossing. Lip biting indicates an attempt to keep information from getting out. Ducking the head between the shoulders in an attempt to hide is called turtling. Squinting diminishes exposure to unwanted knowledge (much like eye-blocking with the hand). Body shifting may occur from general discomfort or from an urge to escape. Shifting eyes may search for escape, or they may meet yours directly, contradicting body-shifting.

Morris cites the hand shrug as a gesture that casts off the person's own words even as they are spoken. Decreased frequency of gesticulation by someone who normally uses their hands while speaking might indicate a degree of exhaustion, or it might indicate repression of any excess or accidental information the hands might relay. Hiding hands behind the back or in pockets to suppress gesticulation may also play a part in alerting you to hidden emotion if you already suspect it. Coin-jingling in pockets is a common sign of general nervousness.

Humans use multiple nonverbal cues due to nerves or distress so the context of the interaction and contradiction between words, body language, and gestures are always key. Navarro makes the important point that if verbal and body signals oppose one another, the truth is most likely found in the negative emotion being revealed.

Human behavior doesn't happen in a vacuum. The same expression or body language that is appropriate in one place may mean something entirely different in another. Navarro emphasizes the importance of a holistic understanding of behavior and the consideration of key contextual elements in reading body language. Here is a simplified formula to help with the process:

- foreknowledge of a person's **baseline behavior** for comparison (this is only possible after repeated interactions)
- **context**: time, place, circumstances, and relationship between actors
- **discrepancies** between verbal and nonverbal communication cues: expression, words, tone, gestures, touch, stance, eye movement, mouth sounds, and proxemics (the use of physical space), as in backing away or moving too close
- **clusters of behaviors** that reinforce one another

Call these BCDC (baseline behavior, context, discrepancies, and clusters of behaviors) to help with memory. Though it may feel a bit like a mathematical equation to keep track of all this, your intuition is already doing a lot of the work. By watching people and cataloging behaviors, you are educating your intuition and making it more efficient.

Verbal Deception

Changing the subject or giving vague or evasive answers is called avoidance. We see this a lot in political debates where questions are ignored, redirected, or turned back on the questioner to avoid a particular subject. Inconsistency is demonstrated when the details of an explanation or story contradict the facts or keep changing over time. A deceptive person may become defensive, even hostile, or may attempt to deflect blame or deny responsibility when questioned about their behavior. You might see a display of anger that is out of proportion to the question asked. A person who responds to an innocuous question with over-the-top anger may be misinterpreting the way an honest person would respond or trying to distract you into changing the subject. Long pauses and disjointed sentences can occur when someone is trying to concoct a story or check their databanks for all the things they said earlier. When people aren't worried about being caught in a lie, they speak freely or even blurt. Some people repeat the question they were asked to buy time. We are told that people who are lying add too many details to a story to make it seem more believable, but people who suffer from impostor syndrome do this as well, so it isn't always a reliable gauge. We are also told to watch for a lack of emotion, since a person attempting to distance themselves from reality may be doing so to avoid giving themselves away. The caveat is that traumatized people may also seem similarly detached.

Just as with nonverbal cues, these cues of verbal deception must be weighed in the moment with the BCDC formula in mind.

Devious Tactics

All warfare is based on deception.
—Sun Tsu, *The Art of War*

Tactics are the small pieces that add up to a greater strategy. When we talk about devious tactics, we are learning to alert ourselves to common yet subtle behaviors that may be used together to gain emotional control over another person. Identify them or be at their mercy.

I'm putting this first installment of devious tactics here, in the intent section, because they are part of a larger process and require time to slowly undermine and weaken the target of abuse (find More Devious Tactics in chapter 7). This is an imperfect science, and these behaviors might be used as part of an interview or positioning strategy as well. Because they are signs of intent that may take time to identify, I have put them here to encourage earliest possible detection.

Common devious and manipulative chronic behaviors to watch for include: guilt-tripping to make you feel you owe something in return; gaslighting, an insidious form of manipulation in which a person with influence in your life denies your reality and emotions in less-than-obvious ways; and negging, a deliberately backhanded compliment meant to undermine your confidence and create a need for the manipulator's validation.

People guilt-trip others to make them feel they owe something in return. Altruistic people will do something because it's right or they enjoy the feeling. Engaging in quid pro quo is petty. Be aware whenever this happens. Scorekeeping is for sports and business, never for personal and social relationships.

Gaslighting systematically causes you to question your perception, memory, even sanity and puts you at the mercy of the abuser's reality. The only important things are the ones the abuser deems so. The only way to live your life is the abuser's way. Any other method of doing things may be met with disdain and you will be told or shown why your thinking is backward. Gaslighting is often done by people who had it done to them and don't know it's abuse, which makes it all the more difficult to identify.

Negging describes someone using backhanded compliments or making deliberately undermining statements such as, "I bet you're really nice to other people." The plan is to keep you from ending the interaction by pressuring you to engage by defending yourself. This tactic keeps you in the game doing what the manipulator wants. The best way to win is not to play. In the longer term negging undermines self-esteem and makes the object of this insidious tactic dependent on the approval of the person doing the negging.

Any or all of these tactics can be used to accomplish the goal of undermining and coercion which weaken self-esteem and agency in any number of ways. Coercion uses intimidation, blackmail, extortion, the threat of physical violence to you or someone you care for, or other underhanded and less obvious threats to cause you to agree to say or do things against your own judgement or will. Some common #MeToo movement examples involve people with power over another person's career and livelihood who force sexual favors in exchange for continued employment.

Grooming is more of a long-term strategy made up of the above tactics. It is most insidious because it involves careful selection of a target based on youth, loneliness, disability, or another vulnerability; the groomer then seeks to emotionally or physically isolate the target from friends and family, gain trust and share "secrets," or to make the relationship feel "special" and therefore exempt from normal rules. The groomer then trains the target to become habituated to various forms of abuse. The way these steps play out is nuanced and should be described early in school so children can learn to identify the subtle signs. As instructors, we should know the specifics of these behaviors and discuss them openly.

If you think someone in your life might be subject to these tactics, or using them against another, interrogate your suspicion or contact RAINN (Rape, Abuse, and Incest National Network) for more information. These tactics may occasionally be employed to force connection between strangers in a bar, but they are most insidious when used early in relationships by those who wish to subjugate and abuse another human being.

Altruism is defined as selfless concern for the welfare of others in order to maintain social connections. No one who engages in the above behaviors is working toward altruistic ends. No matter how kind, gentle, or helpful a person may appear, the use of any one of these behaviors should be an instant red flag. It is your duty to yourself and those who depend on you to recognize the people who employ them. Think of these behaviors as toxic mold or carbon monoxide slowly but inevitably building up in your system.

> ...the verbal attack that is not so grossly obvious and may appear on the surface not to be an attack at all… [is] exceedingly dangerous because so often you don't know they are happening and you therefore make no move to defend yourself. All too often you blame yourself for the havoc they cause in your life.
> —*More on the Gentle Art of Verbal Self-Defense*, by Suzette Haden

Wanting

I see it, I like it, I want it, I got it
I want it, I got it, I want it, I got it, I want it, I got it
I want it, I got it...
—Ariana Grande, from her song "7 Rings"

Wanting is less a direct way to recognize intent than it is a set of emotions that masks our ability to recognize dangerous situations or behaviors. When we want something—to be loved or appreciated, for instance—we often disregard our intuition. Like a child covering the mouth of the sister trying to tell the truth, we unconsciously gag our own best self-protection mechanisms. Remember the story at the beginning of chapter 2 where I let my need to be of service put me in the danger zone? I wanted to do a good deed and that feeling of wanting blinded me to the danger of the unfamiliar place—something that should have been obvious.

People we want things from scramble our signals and we allow them to get too close. Wanting drives cults and peer pressure. We want to be part of a group, to be seen as compatible with others. It's hard to go against the tide because you risk ostracization or worse. In a gang or cult scenario, wanting to fit in can literally save your life.

Sometimes we agree with or buy into something we sense or even know is a bad idea. We want things to be easy, we want to trust, we want good things to be true. Yet nearly every time we want something badly, we are ignoring other important signals.

Desperation and naiveté go hand in hand.
—*Ludwig*, BritBox Original detective series

James Clear, author of *Atomic Habits: An Easy & Proven Way to Build Good Habits & Break Bad Ones*, says researchers have found that 100 percent of the nucleus accumbens is activated when we want something as opposed to only 10 percent when we like something. He says, "Your brain has far more neural circuitry allocated for wanting rewards.... The wanting centers in the brain are large: the ventral tegmental area, the dorsal striatum, the amygdala, and portions of the prefrontal cortex.... They are often referred to as 'hedonic hot spots.'"

Anytime you want something too much, check in with yourself. Make sure your decision-making apparatus is intact, you are paying attention to all your signals, and you aren't just focused on the bling.

> *The planet is shaped by the sheer amazing force of human want, which has changed everything, the forests, the poles, the reservoirs, the glaciers, the rivers, the seas, the mountains, the coast lines, the skies, a planet contoured and landscaped by want.*
> —From *Orbital*, by Samantha Harvey

The Safe Category

A woman I know, let's call her Tina, married a man who later sexually abused her seven-year-old daughter from another marriage. As soon as she began to suspect her new husband, she searched, found clues including child pornography on his computer, and went to the authorities.

Tina's husband went to prison. Though Tina was not able to save her daughter from the initial trauma, she did not turn a blind eye and allow it to continue for years as in another case I know of.

Wanting is not the only way we gag our intuition. When we put people we know in a safe category by thinking, "They would never do that," we blind ourselves to behaviors we deem out of character. I'm not suggesting you begin suspecting friends and family of dirty deeds. I'm suggesting you never disregard your intuition simply because you know someone. There is an additional pressure point with immediate family. Admitting someone we depend on or can't easily avoid is a danger to us or someone close to us presents a very real set of problems that require bravery to acknowledge and address.

Setting Boundaries

Boundary-setting describes the act of creating clear, self-aware rules or markers that define social expectations and protect us from unwanted infringement. This process begins with our understanding of who we are and what makes us comfortable or uncomfortable. We must know what our boundaries are or they won't be clear to others. Learning to set boundaries by early adulthood is crucial, especially for women.

Social boundaries provide everyone with rules about things like respect, distance, and allowances. Your brother probably doesn't shake your hand politely when he sees you, and the mailman doesn't kiss you on the cheek when he drops off your mail. Social behaviors guide us, and we are oblivious to them most of the time. But our obliviousness is what allows smart predators to slip in the door.

Craig: "Have another."
Loni: "I'm good, thanks."
Craig: "Come on, I'm buying."
Loni: "No, really, I'm good, thanks. I don't really want another."
Craig: "I'll have one with you. It's a big day! Let go a little! Really. You're always so hard on yourself. Have a little fun once in a while!"
Loni: "I'll hang out, you have another. I'd love a sparkling water with cranberry, but no more alcohol. I mean it."
Craig: "Jeez! You're no fun. What's your deal!"

Note the subtle yet easily dismissed markers of coercion: negging, cajoling, repeatedly ignoring Loni's no. By implying Loni is uptight, Craig is hoping she will feel the compulsion to contradict him and take the drink. This is one of the ways even unintentionally manipulative people control those who don't like to be labeled or who are anxious to be liked. No one pulled him aside and taught him this. It's an instinct to gain power by putting another on the defensive physically or emotionally.

Craig may be flirting or only want a drinking buddy and the pushing may not be purposeful. Regardless, this sort of behavior should never be taken lightly. A person who will push you to do something you don't want to is likely to do it again. Is this a person who cares whether you have fun? Is this a person who has your welfare in mind? Is this someone you want to drink with? To possibly be drunk with?

Attractive, intelligent, wealthy, or charming predators have an

Chapter 6: The Self-Defense Continuum, Stage 1

advantage. Anytime someone insinuates you are "less than" to make a point or get something from you, it should instantly alert you to a possible agenda. When you are unaware of these devious tactics, anxious to please, or otherwise distracted, you may inadvertently put someone else in control of your decisions and your safety. Don't get stuck on a social script—an exchange of one-liners—where he makes a proposal, you refuse, and the tennis match continues even as you get in his car and hand over control. This person is counting on your concern with social mores to keep you in your place and allow him to maneuver you mentally and physically into his comfort zone and out of yours.

> Kids are excellent boundary pushers. If you're a parent, your kids know your boundaries because they've tested them a thousand times. It's their job to test everyone's boundaries and get as much of what they want as they can. They know exactly how many times they need to push before your "no" becomes a "yes."

Boundaries help you distinguish between someone who abides by social rules and someone who doesn't. When you set boundaries, you demonstrate self-awareness and clarity; when you enforce them, the behavior of those who are comfortable pushing them becomes clear. A person who disregards your clearly set boundaries—who repetitively touches your shoulder in a business relationship that perhaps doesn't call for such intimacy—is telling you they either don't understand boundaries or are disregarding yours outright. This gives you valuable information about that person so you can make decisions accordingly.

Emotional boundary-setting is multi-faceted, but Five Ds of Self-Defense creator Erik Kondo developed a simple tool to illustrate physical boundary-setting by breaking it into three steps. The Progressive Fence consists of the Visual Fence, the Verbal Fence, and the Physical Fence. It's a simple model but simple models are great for making important concepts easy to pass on.

Here's how the Progressive Fence might play out: an acquaintance asks you out and you politely turn him down. He follows you, pleading his case. You stop and hold up both hands—the Visual Fence—and say, "Whoa, enough. I mean it!"—the Verbal Fence. You begin to walk away again but he follows anyway, gesticulating wildly and raising his voice. He may be trying to scare you, he may need to vent, or he may be escalating. You decide not to wait to find out. You get into your car, duck into a store, hail a cab, scream, fight, or several of these measures—the Physical Fence.

These steps illustrate a process we normally take for granted—what we must do to maintain control of an interaction and what the other person does to deny us that control. The more attempts you must make to assert your boundaries, the harder he is trying to deny them. If you make multiple attempts with the Visual and Verbal Fences to no avail, things are escalating. You should already be forming a plan of escape or action.

You probably already use these steps without naming them. The way you use them matters. The body language of the Visual Fence should feel strong. Be sturdy on your feet and keep your hands close in front of your chest. Never stretch your hands out away from your body where they are easy to grab. This position is purposely nonaggressive to avoid escalation. It is also a classic prepared position in many martial arts—hands open in front of your body, on guard, ready to deflect, grab, or attack, which makes it a multi-purpose position. Done properly, the Visual Fence is calm and clear; it is never a challenge or a threat.

The Verbal Fence uses unambiguous and firm but non-threating language: "That's good, ask me from there, thanks." The words "stop" and "no" are important examples of the Verbal Fence and boundary-setting in general. You must never go back once have issued a firm "no" about something you feel strongly about or know is right. Hedging is common, especially among women, and it is a loud, clear sign that differentiates those who know their own minds from those who are willing to bend. Predators are very keyed into this. A person who says "no" two or three times and then ultimately answers "yes" is a person who can be manipulated. A real "no" must never be a negotiation—"Know Your 'No'!" Don't explain or apologize. Change the subject, leave, turn, and speak to someone else. Women often worry about being rude and that is valid. We don't want to piss off the dangerous guy. Devious people depend on this, and they can use it against you. Don't be rude; be

Chapter 6: The Self-Defense Continuum, Stage 1

firm, try deflecting, and saying you have to go to the bathroom. Then disappear.

The responses to your clearly set boundaries are important clues to the kind of person you are interacting with. A social person will stop and shrug at the Visual Fence and go away whereas an asocial person may take it as a challenge. Remember, behavior that will deter a social criminal may attract an asocial one.

If someone consistently ignores your boundaries—whether over minutes or years—be wary. Always pay attention to patterns. If you neglect to enforce your boundaries and allow others to herd you physically or sway you emotionally, you may be setting yourself up as a victim.

Recap

- Before is where we spend most of our time. During, we can only escape, or fight. There are infinite possibilities in the Decide stage, which is about preparation and information gathering.
- Intent implies commitment and willingness to undertake risk. Pay attention to signals from your intuition: inarticulable doubt, nagging feelings, suspicion, hesitation, and true fear, among other signals.
- Situational awareness refers to the ability to perceive multiple elements in a dynamic environment, comprehend the ways in which they interact, and project potential problems. We can cultivate enhanced perception using Amy Herman's four As—assess, analyze, articulate, and adapt (as explained in her book *Visual Intelligence*) and by engaging in challenging visual attention tasks.
- Nonverbal deception includes facial expressions, gestures, touch, stance, eye contact and movement, and mouth sounds.
    - o Try to articulate the differences between similar emotions like surprise and fear or anger, disgust, and contempt.
    - o Micro-expressions last a fifteenth or twenty-fifth of a second and are accidental leaks that display concealed emotion or intention.
    - o Autonomic signals from physiological changes beyond conscious control are most difficult to mask: fast breathing, sweating, excessive or arrested blinking, dry mouth, and pupil dilation.

- o Consider key contextual elements in reading body language. BCDC reminds us to account for *baseline behaviors* for comparison, *context* (time, place, and relationship), *discrepancies* between verbal and nonverbal cues, and *clusters of behaviors*.
- o Lie detection is unreliable, though lying does use more energy and focus, which can cause contradictions between verbal and physical cues. Catching a lie and calling a person out may cause a backlash regardless of who is right.
  - Some people lack function in areas of the brain that differentiate between lies and truth and don't display as many tells.
  - Joe Navarro says if verbal and body language signals oppose each other, the truth is often in the negative emotion being revealed.
- Verbal deception: avoidance, inconsistency, defensiveness, long pauses, and disjointed sentences. Repeating the question to buy time. People who suffer from impostor syndrome may add too many details to a story, so it may not be a reliable gauge. The same goes for lack of emotion—traumatized people may also seem similarly detached.
- Devious tactics: tactics are small pieces that add up to a strategy: guilt-tripping, gaslighting, negging, undermining, coercion, intimidation, blackmail, extortion, and threats of physical violence. Grooming is an insidious, long-term strategy made up of multiple tactics that involves careful selection of a target based on youth, loneliness, disability, or another vulnerability.
- Wanting is less a direct way to recognize intent than it is a set of emotions that masks our ability to do so. When we want something, we often disregard our intuition.
- When we put trusted people in the safe category by thinking, "They would never do that," we may blind ourselves to behaviors we would ordinarily notice.
- **Setting Boundaries** helps you distinguish between someone who abides by social rules and someone who doesn't. It involves setting realistic limits on interactions to protect yourself from unwanted infringement. Learning this by early adulthood is crucial, especially for women.

- o Exhibit clear, consistent behavior and stand by it.
- o Social boundaries provide everyone with rules about respect, distance, and allowances.
- o A person who will push you to do something you don't want to is likely to do so again.
- o Attractive, intelligent, wealthy, or charming predators have an advantage.
- o Erik Kondo's Progressive Fence consists of the Visual Fence, the Verbal Fence, and the Physical Fence.

Suggested Practice

 I've seen this exercise in several places. Emily Fletcher of Ziva Meditation calls it Come to Your Senses. Rory Miller calls it Centering and says he picked it up from a manual on psychological first aid to calm traumatized children. This exercise brings you into your body in the present moment and connects you with all five senses. Mindfulness exercises like this can pave the road to a stronger connection with your intuition. I often just use the first three of the five parts of the exercise. Find someplace safe and comfortable and close your eyes for five or ten minutes.

- **Note a few things you hear.** Loud, soft, close, far away. Don't judge any of it.
- **Note a few things you see** through closed eyelids: the visual static, the light, the dark, whatever was in front of you before, or a calming place of your choosing.
- **Note a few things you smell.** Don't judge, just smell as you breathe. Nothing or just air is fine.
- **Note a few things you feel.** Your body against the chair. The pillows. The breeze. Your feet on the floor.
- **Note a few things you taste.** Do you taste toothpaste? Your last meal? Or nothing at all, which is fine too.

CHAPTER 7

The Self-Defense Continuum, Stage 2—Deter the Interview

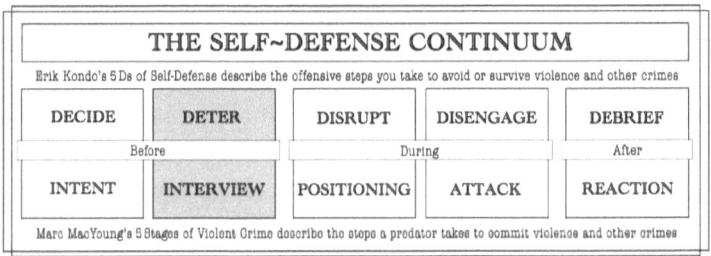

SDC Stage 2: Deter/Interview

An ounce of prevention is worth a pound of cure.
    —Benjamin Franklin

In the last chapter on recognizing criminal intent, I told a story about how I avoided a man soliciting in an empty parking lot while my toddler was in the back seat of our car. It worked there as an illustration of stacked behaviors setting off my intuition, but it also works here to illustrate what it looks like in real time to Deter at the Interview stage. My intuition lit up (intent recognition) and I drove away (interview deterrence). It's hardly a story of courage and bravery in the face of extreme danger. I simply avoided a situation that made me uncomfortable. Doing this won't win you fanfare or medals. It won't leave you with an anecdote you can recount over and over. Yawn. You also won't have a story to tell from the hospital or the psychiatrist's office.

Assuming we've recognized criminal intent, what do we do next? Since we don't want to engage further with anyone who might intend us harm, we need to deter him from learning more about us and becoming any more invested in his plan. We need to fail his interview by being too troublesome or dangerous (smart, prepared, supported by others) to bother with. The Twelve Traits of Protective Offense supply you with a dozen ways to fail an interview.

> *Ultimate victory is in avoiding the fight.*
> —Sun Tzu

In the movie *Enter the Dragon*, Bruce Lee famously illustrates the concept of fighting without fighting: when challenged by a boastful opponent, Lee persuades him to step off a crowded boat onto a small rowboat so they can go to an island where there will be more room to fight. He then unties the rowboat, leaving his opponent stranded. The scene is a wonderful visual example of the philosophy that true martial arts mastery is less about physical prowess than the ability to outthink and outmaneuver opponents.

We know what it means to deter someone, but what is a criminal interview and what does it look like? Do the two of you sit down and chat? Possibly. Or it could look like a chance encounter, a plea for help, or even a date. The interview is any process a predator uses to observe and choose a victim. This can be done from up close or far away and can take minutes or months depending on the type of crime. Generally, a criminal needs to make sure of two things: that you have what he wants and that it's safe for him to attack you without being injured or captured. The more determined or invested an attacker, the less he may be worried about injury or capture, but these are usually part of his equation.

If a criminal contacts you by phone, text, or social media, he will need to arrange a face-to-face interview, unless he is engaging in a cyber-attack. Our primary concentration is on violent crime, but if he wants you to transfer funds, the interview, positioning, and attack stages can happen over the internet without a meeting ever needing to occur.

In a crime of opportunity—say, a purse snatching—the interview might involve a criminal scanning the crowd for a dangling purse and finding you distracted by your phone. The way you deter this interview is in the decide stage where you've made an effort to be actively aware.

With a stalking—a longer-term interview—someone might watch you over days or months. Even here, deterrence involves being actively aware and using knowledge from previous chapters to present yourself as a hard target. If you make it too dangerous for him to proceed—if he feels you will fight back or catch him before he completes his plan—he may well move on.

The more determined and devious a criminal, the more complicated the interview. Hone your intuition. Whenever these signals light up, you should pay attention. If you are in an unfamiliar or sketchy area, this is even more urgent. But what constitutes a sketchy area?

On the Fringe

> *You look at these scattered houses and you are impressed by their beauty. I look at them and the only thought which comes to me is a feeling of their isolation and of the impunity with which crime may be committed there.*
> —From *The Complete Stories of Sherlock Holmes Volume I*, by Sir Arthur Conan Doyle

Most of this book is less about knowing everything than asking the right questions. You cannot, however, ask questions you don't know are available to you, so a lot depends on learning what those are. Criminals are intimately familiar with society's fringe and we are not. They are like fish looking up at insects on the surface of the water. They are in their comfort zone. You can see them but only if you know what to look for.

For this reason we need to be familiar with all the nuances of these violence-prone places. Fringe areas are places where things happen because they can. That's a bit vague, but it helps me to think of it that simply.

These are places that lack resources: light, people, exits. They tend to be unpopulated places outside main public thoroughfares—places on the periphery or on the way to and from somewhere else: hallways, stairways, shortcuts, elevators, alleys, garages, train yards, loading areas, parking structures. Your own home can be a fringe area in the case of domestic violence or a home invasion. The inside of a house is secluded and private, the way we like it when we shower and sleep. But criminals like privacy too. A place might be on the fringe because it's silent and deserted and no one is around to hear you, or because it's too noisy for you to be heard. A public restroom or room of a house during a party can be on the fringe because no one outside can hear you. Fringe areas can also be temporary or transient. An office building might only be on the fringe after hours. Violence often occurs in bars and clubs with lots of people around. So, we must add that the fringe is also any place people go to get drunk or high. I've heard it said, "If people can see you or hear you but can't reach you, or could reach you *if* they could see or hear you, you are in a fringe area."

Anything unusual or discomfiting that happens in a fringe area should immediately alert your intuition simply because it's a fringe area. If a stranger approaches you in a fringe area for any reason, keep your distance and insist the other person keep theirs. Use the Progressive Fence. Most socially aware people understand a woman's position in the world. Only someone who is desperate, oblivious, or who has an agenda will expect a woman to stand still as he approaches her in an unpopulated place. This behavior alone should be enough to cause your guard to activate. In this, as in many things, ego gets in the way. We don't want to appear weak or fearful so we hide our concern. Never allow a stranger to infringe (pun intended) on your comfort zone out of politeness.

Because the fringe can be complicated, it's important to ask the right questions: Do I know where I am? Am I prepared to be here? What resources do I have with me: phone, people, weapons, running shoes, car? Could help arrive within a few minutes? Try to recognize when you're in a fringe area as early as possible and keep your guard up while you're there. You might even consider keeping a weapon of some sort in hand or in your pocket until you get to a less fringy place (we'll talk more about weapons in subsequent chapters).

> Some people carry fringe areas with them. They are invisible to others even in broad daylight on crowded streets. Teenagers harassing other teenagers will often go unnoticed unless their antics affect others. The unhoused, the poor, queer folks, and black and brown people will often be ignored even when terrible things occur. In many cases, just being in these categories attracts danger from multiple sources. This is a whole different issue, but it bears consideration. Empathetic, informed bystanders are urgently needed in these cases.

Marc MacYoung's Five Interview Strategies

According to Marc MacYoung, there are five interview strategies: regular, hot, escalating, silent, and prolonged.

A regular interview consists of a criminal approaching you to express a need: the time, a cigarette, directions. This is his way of distracting you while also checking your awareness and commitment to defending yourself. If, when he approaches, you are too busy with your phone to look up, or you appear lost, or your bag is dangling, he may grab it and run.

This is the most common interview type for muggers, but rapists also use it. This interview might also be used by teams where one criminal pretending to be distracted and desperately lost distracts you while his accomplice grabs your bag.

I was fourteen on a crowded city street when a guy in front of me suddenly began limping. I immediately sensed bad acting and was moving to his side to get a better view when I felt a hand in my bag. I spun quickly and both prospective thieves ran off empty-handed. As a born-and-bred city girl, I never carried anything of value in accessible places anyway. I remember shaking my head as I crossed Times Square before it was shiny and new. Active awareness may be enough to deter a regular interview.

The hot interview is a sudden, often loud, out-of-nowhere, mind-jarring emotional bombardment. One minute you're doing your thing, the next you're facing a threatening, obscenity-spouting human-shaped monster. MacYoung says, "The success of this strategy relies on you not being accustomed to dealing with extreme emotional violence and reacting in a stunned and confused manner." A stunned victim is an easy victim. The hot interview is a tried-and-true strategy for a criminal team. The hot interview guy distracts you with harsh language while an accomplice robs you.

If you live in a city, you may have encountered this type of behavior from someone who is drunk or high, though it may not have been an interview, just a person in trouble, venting. Knowing the difference can be difficult and usually has to do with other signals or the amount of anger directed at you and not just at the air. People with goals tend to be focused.

There is no need to stick around to decipher this behavior. If anyone comes at you raving, exit stage left. Don't worry about what you look like scampering away. Do you want your headstone to read, "At least she didn't die of embarrassment"?

The escalating interview is a hybrid of the previous two and rapidly goes from regular to hot. Imagine a normal encounter with a stranger that suddenly turns hostile. This is what it looks like when a criminal tests your boundaries. He may continue to escalate—sometimes very quickly—until his behavior becomes physical.

The silent interview describes a criminal observing you for enough time to accumulate details that make him feel proprietary about you or that supply him with knowledge about your habits or your possessions. What he needs to know might only take a few moments, depending on the intended crime. This predator goes through the Intent and Interview stages without any direct interaction with you, which means you may never have a face-to-face encounter until he positions himself for the attack.

The prolonged interview can take days, weeks, or longer. With prolonged interviews, the criminal's intent isn't always obvious. Stalkers are the most obvious prolonged interviewers. A rapist might engage in a silent prolonged interview, watching his victim for days or more without ever interacting. A scam artist might use a regular prolonged interview, where he chats you up to gain your trust over a period of days or more.

It will take all the skill sets in this book to recognize intent and deter the silent or prolonged interview.

More Devious Tactics

Victimizers can use devious tactics at many stages of the SDC, and we mentioned several in chapter 6 when we discussed Intent. You may remember that these include but are not limited to guilt-tripping, gas-lighting, negging, undermining, coercion, intimidation, blackmail, extortion, threat of physical violence, and grooming. Look up these words and terms and familiarize yourself not just with what they mean, but how they look and feel. Do they bring up any familiar scenarios great or small?

There are too many tactics to mention, some with no names because creative criminals synthesize them on the spot. We've discussed what it means to "Know Your 'No'" earlier in the section on boundary-setting. This involves a troublemaker testing the strength or flexibility of your most urgent boundaries.

"No" is one of the first words we learn as children and most parents are familiar with the "no" stage of development where this wonderful new word is regularly exercised to show autonomy and control over personal boundaries. It's a very important (though annoying) stage and, though not every childhood "no" is reasonable, "nos" should be honored by parents with questions rather than demands whenever possible. Sometimes our "no" weakens as we grow into adult social life and seek to please and maintain the peace.

Sometimes using the word "no" hurts feelings and causes escalation of emotion. "No, thank you" is sometimes better than just "no." Deflection or little white lies are valid ways to turn someone down gently without explicitly saying "no." "I'll think about it" is one deflection. "I have plans, maybe next time" is a little white lie and a deflection that allows a potentially unstable person to save face, something we will discuss shortly. These are more subtle forms of "no," but they are still "nos" in the moment.

Any clear, firm "no" should be the end of negotiations. Anyone who disregards your decisive "no" is telling you they don't respect you and they have an agenda—one that benefits them, not you.

If you're feeling uneasy about an interaction and want to know if a person respects your personal agency, instructor and author Shihan Michelle suggests two tactics. Try a testing "no" to something he proposes and see how he reacts. His response will supply you with important information about future interactions. You might also try a counteroffer. Shihan Michelle gives the example of refusing to give your own phone number and asking for his instead. The counteroffer is a "no" with a softening caveat. Asocial people may have more trouble accepting this than social ones.

"Don't WE on ME!" Another tactic is abuse of the word "we." "We" may be used by a criminal to ingratiate himself and get closer to you by implying something you both have in common. When strangers use the word "we" to describe you both as one, they are implying a relationship. This is fine if you're both in line for a movie and the "we" stops there. If it becomes a way to push the boundaries of trust it's a problem. Trust is valuable. It should never be rushed or given out of courtesy or carelessness.

We often hear about what I call the Liar's Litany—when liars use extra detail to shore up their stories. Where the truth sounds straightforward—"Sorry, traffic. Left late. My bad."—lying goes long, "There was this accident between a red Mercedes—really nice car"—blah, blah, blah—"I think someone died … that's why I was so late." Sometimes the extra details feel off, sometimes they don't. Our understanding of verbal and nonverbal signals within a context can help us sort this kind of thing out in the moment.

The important caveat here is that people on the autism or ADHD spectrum, those with low self-esteem who feel chronically doubted, and people who suffer from imposter syndrome, also sometimes give more details than necessary when making excuses.

Charm or Harm? Many conflict analysts will talk about charm, which is not an inherent trait but a social strategy to get people to like you, hire you, or do things for you. The word suggests a magical element that is backed up by its synonyms: enchant, bewitch, entrance, enthrall. We are naturally more alert to bad behavior so charm takes us by surprise and disarms our natural intuitive processes, and criminals know it. We will dodge a punch, but not a compliment.

> *Demons will charm you with a smile . . .*
> —From *Sweeny Todd*

The Gift of Fear is indispensable to anyone who wants to be able to identify other specific tactics commonly used by criminals. Author Gavin de Becker speaks at length about charm and several other urgent indicators of criminal intent or ulterior motives he calls pre-incident indicators or PINS in this seminal work.

These predatory tactics busy you defending rather than taking initiative and blind you to the intentions of a potential perpetrator. They should immediately alert your intuition. Why would a stranger be trying to get under your skin or inside your guard? There must be a reason, and it may not be altruistic. That said, not everyone who uses these tactics is a deviant or criminal. Ask yourself if you ever use these tactics. How do you respond to "no"? We are all human and tend to use what we have to get what we want unless our conscience and ethics stop us. Don't judge people overly harshly. Use what you are learning to spot groups of signals, then look deeper to see if more is going on.

Deter by De-escalation

> *It is better to avoid than to run, better to run than to de-escalate, better to de-escalate than to fight, better to fight than to die.*
> —Rory Miller, *Facing Violence: Preparing for the Unexpected*

My father-in-law was pushing his cart through a hardware store when a younger cart-wielding man rammed into him. The younger man shouted and demanded an apology. My father-in-law listened patiently, allowing the man to vent, then leaned in and said, "I'm so sorry, I'm getting older and I don't see or hear so well anymore." The younger man dissolved on the spot and apologized profusely for his behavior.

Often, when someone loses their temper, we get sucked in and mirror emotion, throwing gasoline on the fire. High emotion escalates the odds of catastrophe. De-escalation starves the fire of oxygen. It requires us to avoid being infected with the other person's emotion even though that's what we are designed for.

> *I don't got a short fuse, you just don't know when you lit it!*
> —Bill Murray, *The Greatest Beer Run Ever*

Remember that social crime is for socially motivated purposes: status within a group, team, family, or gang. A crime of reeducation might begin with, "I told you to do it, now do it!" or "I'm in charge here." Gang violence is brutal but socially motivated, and so is domestic violence. Asocial crimes are the domain of predators who see you as subhuman. Predators hunt; they don't respond to normal social cues. Both social and asocial people can become violent, but asocial predators are harder to spot. This is where de-escalation indirectly does a great service. A person who doesn't respond to your de-escalation strategy may be notifying you of their asocial tendencies.

If a social person is agitated for social reasons (they just lost their job) de-escalation can save time, trouble, and teeth. Active listening techniques work well: speaking in open-ended sentences to draw out details, nodding or using other forms of encouragement like humming ("mm-hmm…"), paraphrasing what was just said so the speaker feels heard, mirroring some of the speaker's emotion, and summarizing what was said to show you listened.

De-escalation nearly always includes speaking calmly, clearly, and slowly and in your lowest tone. It may include commiserating, appeasing, and other similar social skills so long as they are non-patronizing. If you don't actually care, you risk slipping into the annoyed parent role. Once he sees you are only in it to end it, he is unlikely to give you another chance.

As a rule, de-escalation only works with social criminals. Verbal de-escalation sometimes has a detrimental effect on communication with asocial people. A loud and clear "I said no!" when there are people nearby might be the only caveat. "No" is not a threat, insult, or challenge—things we will talk more about in a moment. Though it is a command, it is not a command that they do something controversial like relax or calm down, which I consider four-letter words. Shouting is generally contraindicated, but if there are people around, saying "no" loudly might be effective. Predators tend to prefer doing their business in the shadows. Say "no" loudly, say it clearly, and do not qualify it or answer questions. Put your hands up in a double-stop position (the Visual Fence) but do not stretch them out and offer them up. Maintain your distance, do not engage him in conversation, and do not give in to social impulses. You are telling him you see him and are aware of what he is doing. If you resort to social behaviors, he will call your bluff.

By the time a predator chooses you, you have already been othered. Trying to talk him out of it, flattering him, and commiserating with him about how the world sucks and you are on his side are all social answers to social altercations. Use these strategies with your drunk friend who you know well. Use them in a safe environment. Trying to connect in a human way like mentioning your kids waiting for you at home may be seen as weakness that could excite him and trigger the chase instinct. Don't show your throat. Play your cards close to the vest and don't give away information or babble. Don't escalate emotion by insulting, challenging, threatening, or commanding.

Peyton Quinn's Rules of Escalation-Avoidance

Reality-based self-defense pioneer Peyton Quinn came up with five simple yet profoundly important ways to avoid escalating a potentially violent altercation, and security expert Richard Dimitri added a sixth. These fundamental rules apply to any situation involving an angry, unstable individual: do not insult him, do not challenge him, do not threaten him, do not command him (Dimitri's addition), do not deny it's happening, but do give him a face-saving exit.

The first four could be grouped into: do not insult, challenge, threaten, or command him. These are similar and have the same effect of forcing a response from someone on the edge of anger or violence. To these I would add the obvious: do not shout at him.

Let's save Quinn's last two stand-alone rules for later and put the first four together with my addition. If we juggle the order a bit: do not shout, threaten, insult, challenge, command, we get the acronym STICC—unwieldy as acronyms go but easier to remember and refer to.

Don't STICC it to him: Do not shout, threaten, insult, challenge, or command. These are often reflexive responses to emotion that overwhelms us. Though there are similarities, each of these has its own particular flavor.

Shouting raises emotion, no matter what you're saying. We can threaten, insult, challenge, and command without shouting. Shouting makes it worse. The only caveat is once again the loud-and-clear "Stop!," "No!," or "Don't touch me!," generally with enough people around to make it more difficult for the troublemaker to follow through.

We use threats when we feel cornered and can't think of anything else to do. A threat is a mask of desperation.

We use insults when we forget how to use other words. Insults are emotions bubbling over. The sounds and syllables of most curses and insults are sharp and emotionally satisfying, but they make problems rather than solve them.

Challenges are dangerous games of one-upmanship. If you don't want to raise the stakes, don't use challenging language. If you do, be prepared for him to call your bluff. "What are you going to do? Shoot

Chapter 7: The Self-Defense Continuum, Stage 2

us?" This is purportedly how a young New York City actress named Nicole DuFresne challenged her shooter. They were her last words.

> Nicole DuFresne, her fiancé, and two friends were mugged by seven teens in the early hours on the Lower East Side of Manhattan. One gun-wielding teen pistol-whipped DuFresne's fiancé during a mugging. DuFresne's fiancé reportedly said, "Let's just go," as one of their friends helped him up. DuFresne then walked up on the gun-wielding mugger and challenged him with those final words. *The New York Times* reported on the testimony of one of the muggers, saying it was DuFresne's "attitude, defiance, and disdain" that caused the nineteen-year-old, first-time mugger to shoot her dead.

When we challenge someone with an unstable ego, we are in a way forcing their hand. We are saying, "Back down!" And criminals, especially, are not in the habit of doing this.

A lack of physical strength may cause us to overcompensate with verbal abuse when we aren't prepared for the violence that can cause.

We command when we feel small and need to regain a feeling of power. This is interesting when you consider that another word for command is order, and an order is usually only given by someone with authority: a parent to a child, a boss to a worker, a sergeant to an enlisted grunt. To a disenfranchised person who lacks power in the social world, an order adds insult to injury. A command or order may alert the same response as a violent attack and therefore demand an immediate and sometimes catastrophic response.

To STICC it to anyone virtually guarantees escalation. Never fool yourself that you can get away with shouting, insulting, challenging, or commanding someone without some sort of backlash. After an emotional outburst, we mostly rationalize or do damage control. Ego is a huge driver of detrimental emotional decision-making. It's important to check the bigger picture and the emotions behind our behavior. The top dog, or alpha, is usually the quietest and least challenging one in the pack. He doesn't need to make a big fuss.

Impulse control is an extremely underrated skill. There is no easy way to hack into lightning-fast, knee-jerk emotional signals from our limbic system (monkey brain). Cognitive and dialectic behavioral modalities have had success over lengthy periods, but good practitioners are elusive and expensive. In the meantime, we are left to scrounge for our own individual answers.

One suggestion is to try a little time travel. Imagine, for a moment, that you are confronted by an enraged ex-lover. Your ego wants to assert itself; the pressure to say what's on your mind is overwhelming. Perhaps a vision of the worst-possible outcome might help you hold your tongue. When it comes to violent people, do you want to be right or do you want to live? Is the last word worth your last breath?

Quinn's last two stand-alone rules are:

- **Do Not Deny It's Happening:** So much goes wrong because we refuse to believe that this thing is happening to us. What begins with simple denial can become a kind of mind freeze as the situation escalates. We are still there, blinking, perhaps moving, or talking, but the part of our brain that recognizes and deals with danger has frozen.

  The "this can't be happening" response is common and even more insidious when we are familiar with the perpetrator. Remember this quote from Lt. Col Dave Grossman: "It is difficult to believe and accept that anyone we like and identify with is capable of [horrific] acts against their fellow human beings.... This simple naive tendency is possibly, more than any other factor, responsible for the perpetuation of atrocity and horror in our world today."
  If you find yourself wondering if something is really happening, it probably is.

- **Provide Him with a Face-Saving Exit:** Faced with a loud, irrational, and possibly unhinged personality, you might consider choosing to back down first using phrases like, "I see your point" or "I was out of line." Make sure you use a nonconfrontational tone, or it may negate your words.

You might try a tactical apology, even if he's wrong. If it doesn't work, you may be dealing with an asocial individual who doesn't recognize the social value of apology. This should immediately notify you to change your strategy.

Providing a volatile individual with an honorable exit makes it easier for him to disengage without feeling like a coward or loser. Beware: your ego may do everything to stop you. You will need to relinquish the need to make your point or have the last word. This may require some fairly complex emotional acrobatics. It can feel like trying to stop yourself while rolling down a steep hill. When it comes to fast-twitch anger and frustration responses, self-awareness practices are first and foremost.

It can be even more difficult afterward not to dwell on the decision to back down and feel you made the weak choice. Assertiveness can be accomplished in many ways. Counterintuitively, the louder the assertion the less assertive it is. Give yourself credit for being the bigger, quieter dog.

> A coworker of my husband's once successfully escaped a disturbing coffee shop stalker without confrontation. At first, she was relieved, but when she told her boss, he said she should have taken control—stood her ground and told the guy to back off. She spent weeks feeling stupid for not having done more, even though confronting him would have violated the STICC rule. Often potentially well-meaning yet inexperienced people give us advice intended to empower us that instead leaves us feeling weak. Trying to win a battle with an unhinged person is never a useful strategy. Ask yourself what a confrontation might have led to. Don't waste time wondering if you—as Rory Miller once put it—"survived wrong." Pat yourself on the back, regroup, and move on.

Recap

- The interview stage is the process of a predator observing and choosing a victim.
- Unusual behavior in fringe areas should immediately alert our intuition because crimes that happen there may happen faster and with more violence than they would in other places.

- Marc MacYoung gave us five interview types: regular, hot, escalating, silent, and prolonged.
- More devious tactics include: Know Your "No," Don't WE on ME!, The Liar's Litany, and Charm or Harm.
- Deter by de-escalation and starve the fire of oxygen. Be an active listener. Use open-ended sentences to draw out details, nod, hum encouragement ("mm-hmm…"), paraphrase or summarize what was just said to show understanding, mirror the speaker's emotion, speak calmly, clearly, slowly and in your lowest tone. Commiserate or appease so long as you don't patronize.
  o Verbal de-escalation skills have a limited and sometimes detrimental effect on communication with asocial people. A loud and clear "I said No!" when there are people nearby might be the only caveat.
  o Peyton Quinn's Rules of Escalation-Avoidance (with embellishments): Don't STICC it to him: Do not shout, threaten, insult, challenge, or command. Quinn's crucial two final rules are:
    ▪ Do not deny it's happening.
    ▪ Provide him with a face-saving exit.

Suggested Practices

 On the Fringe: Name potential fringe areas as you see them. What makes them fringe areas? Ask yourself how long it would take for anyone to notice you or come to your aid. If the answer is more than a few minutes, catalogue your resources and make a plan.

 STICCy Business. Ever STICC it to someone then wonder why things went sideways? Think, write, or dictate about a time you lost control and escalated a situation—a time you shouted, commanded, challenged, threatened, or insulted someone. It hurts, I know. Your ego will tell you this is dumb. Do it anyway. Dig in to the discomfort. Dissect it. Think about how it felt and why you couldn't stop yourself from rushing toward the last word.

What could you have done differently? Could you perhaps have used your new deescalation skills? Or take a page out of Chapter 2 and reframed the situation? Taken on the persona of someone you respected and behaved the way they would have? Connected to the other person's reality? Or projected an outcome that would have made you proud?

How would things have changed? What would it have felt like to have responded rather than reacted? Be willing to examine and tinker with your own emotional triggers to understand what might trigger others.

CHAPTER 8

The Self-Defense Continuum, Stage 3— Disrupt Positioning

THE SELF~DEFENSE CONTINUUM				
Erik Kondo's 5 Ds of Self-Defense describe the offensive steps you take to avoid or survive violence and other crimes				
DECIDE	DETER	DISRUPT	DISENGAGE	DEBRIEF
Before		During		After
INTENT	INTERVIEW	POSITIONING	ATTACK	REACTION
Marc MacYoung's 5 Stages of Violent Crime describe the steps a predator takes to commit violence and other crimes				

SDC Stage 3: Disrupt/Positioning

Every step forward along the Continuum removes opportunities. The Positioning stage presents the last opportunity to escape a potentially violent encounter by nonviolent means. The next stage—Attack—moves you from Before to During on the Self-Defense Continuum and forces you into physicality.

The positioning stage is where a criminal meets you or maneuvers you into a place or situation that gives him the upper hand. To complicate matters, interview and positioning can blur into a single moment. A threat engages you in a hot interview—he charges you down, spewing epithets—and in the process backs you into a doorway. How you respond to being charged down is the irecap the pnterview, but if it works, he's already got you in position.

On other occasions, the interview and positioning stages might be more spread out, which affords you a bit more time. Remember that there is always less time when you are in a fringe area.

Never let the enemy pick the battle site.
—General Patton

Marc MacYoung's Five Positioning Strategies

Marc MacYoung's Five Positioning Strategies are the most common documented strategies criminals use to get close to their victims. They are: closing, cornering, surprise, split, and surrounding. It may help you to remember that they begin with two Cs and three Ss.

The first strategy, called closing, as in closing distance, mirrors MacYoung's regular interview, which we discussed in the previous chapter. In closing, as in the regular interview, a potential criminal approaches you in need of something like a light or directions. That's it. The need gets him close to you. Here, the interview and positioning stages can sometimes blur, and what begins as an interview leads directly to positioning.

Cornering (or trapping) is a positioning strategy in which a criminal traps you between himself and a large object or where he blocks the exit. Always try to exercise active awareness when you are in unfamiliar places. Note multiple exits; don't depend on a single one. Don't corner yourself by heading into unknown areas or down one-way access points. These are important habits to build. I find this to be a good I Spy-type game with young kids. How many exits or ways in or out can you find in this movie theater, library, or school?

Chapter 8: The Self-Defense Continuum, Stage 3

The surprise strategy is the ambush. It's that "holy crap!" moment of the movie where the guy appears in the back seat of the car or the closet and you don't see him until it's too late. You can avoid many ambush types with active awareness.

If you were going to jump out and surprise a friend, where would you hide? Thought exercises supply insight into how someone might use the environment against you.

Watch for easy hiding spots and give them a wide berth when you're alone—bushes, trees, cars. Walk down the middle of the block so you are never within arm's reach of doorways or vehicles. Watch for predators hidden in plain sight. As in nature, predators use camouflage. A predator might wear clothing that blends in with buildings or wear black or dark gray at night. If a thing blends in and doesn't move, even if it's in front of us, we often don't see it. Use your peripheral vision to track movement, color, and pattern by softening your gaze so you see a wide angle. This turns your eyes into motion sensors. Have your keys ready before you get to your car or door—don't stand with your back to the rest of the world fumbling in your bag. Check the back seat of your car before getting in. Use reflective surfaces like windows and car mirrors to see behind you while unlocking doors or looking in shop windows. Keep a weapon ready in hand (see sidebar), especially in fringe areas.

> You can buy pepper spray and hard or pointy trinkets that serve as protective weapons to clip to your keys. We rarely go anywhere without our keys. You can even simply carry the pointiest key (usually a car key) sticking out—not from between your first two fingers, as is most often taught—but from the pinky side of your hand (the figure below shows a key held in hammer-fist). The skin is not so delicate, which makes it easier to hold on to, and there is more you can do with it from that position (more in chapter 9). If you don't have a car key you can buy a blank and add it to your key ring, though there are other options on the market. Almost any hard object you can comfortably hold onto is better than nothing. Have your weapon in hand whenever the situation calls for extra caution. If you need to fumble through all the junk in your purse to find your go-to item, you may as well not have it at all.

Reimagining Women's Self-Defense

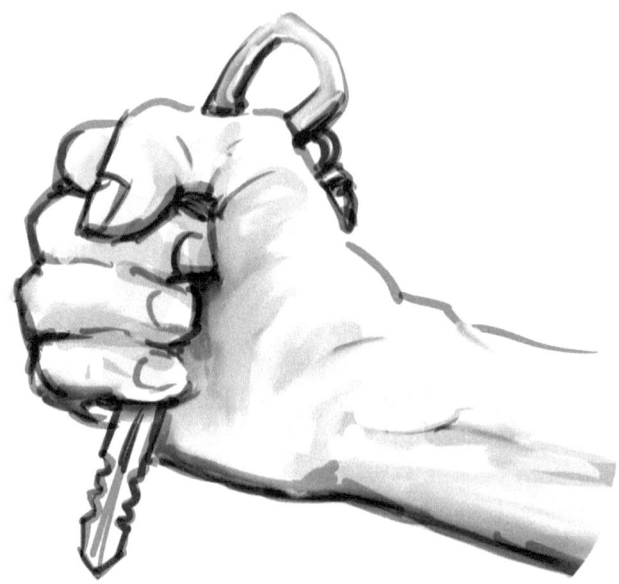

How to hold a key for protection

The next positioning strategy is known as split (or sometimes pincer). We know that criminals sometimes work in teams or gangs and split is an effective strategy when they do. Active or situational awareness can thwart this strategy. Notice your surroundings, odd or deliberate behavior, changes in your environment. Don't walk into a trap. Never walk through people standing apart but appearing to be together and watching others covertly. Cross the street or take a detour around them.

Split takes several forms:
- Two or more people suddenly split up as they approach you. You might have seen kids do this to harass or bully another kid. It's highly disconcerting to engage several people at once, one of whom may be behind you or to the side.
- One thug engages you from the front using the closing strategy, and the other blindsides you or grabs your bag. (This is what happened to me when I was fourteen in Times Square, as I recounted earlier.)

Chapter 8: The Self-Defense Continuum, Stage 3

- Two guys face each other across a narrow walkway so you have no choice but to walk between them.

The fifth strategy is surrounding, which involves at least three people. It's a more complex version of split in which you walk by or through a group and are suddenly surrounded. They may swarm quickly to overwhelm you or drift so they have time to read you.

When I was about eleven, a group of girls closed in around me and demanded my money in broad daylight on a crowded street very close to my house. I gave them my little yellow wallet. No one on the street was even aware anything was going on. People flowed around us like water. We were just a bunch of kids doing kid things that didn't concern them. It was particularly shocking at the time since I was in a place I considered safe, not a fringe area, not dark, not deserted. I was invisible because I was a kid with other kids. Had I yelled, someone might have stepped up, but I was in shock and embarrassed, and I froze—something we will talk more about shortly.

Being aware of these strategies makes them easier to spot and gives you notice so you can remove yourself before they progress to the next stage.

Nonviolent Disruption at the Positioning Stage

Your assailant has invested time and energy and is determined to get what he came for. If he has othered you, appeals to his humanity will fail. I've heard people recommend vomiting or acting crazy, but I have yet to meet anyone who can vomit on command, and the mentally ill and handicapped are high-risk groups, which could mean bodily functions won't be a reliable crime deterrent.

Violence is always an option, so be ready to launch into explosive action and pull out all the stops. But once you attack him, you give him permission to do the same, so be sure it is the only option.

Make Like a Tree

> *Why don't you make like a tree and get outta here!*
> —Ad-libbed by Thomas F. Wilson ("Biff"), *Back to the Future*

The positioning stage is where you haven't yet been attacked but suspect you're in the wrong place with the wrong person. This is your last chance to avoid physicality. Don't wait. If possible, walk, run, make like a tree, and leave. Leaving is one of the best violence-avoidance strategies. It's difficult to get into trouble if you're not there. This may mean playing along, making an excuse that you need to go to the bathroom then disappearing, moving to a safer location, or simply running.

Your best option is always to escape, but only if he won't see you, can't outrun you, or there is a safe location within sprinting distance. Running away is a legitimate, honorable, and even a recommended self-defense technique, but you should be able to depend on your ability in a pinch. Don't expect to run well because you ran twenty years ago in school. I was shocked at how easy it was for my fourteen-year-old son to outrun me. It was quite a reality check. Don't count on a skill unless it's tested. If you plan to use running as a protective tactic, you don't have to train for the Olympics, but you might consider practicing sprints. See how quickly you can take off against someone bigger or taller than you. Short bursts of ten to thirty seconds will do. Sprints are an effective and efficient cardio exercise, so when you practice you can skip the treadmill.

Remember, you will be under stress. Adrenaline doesn't always make you faster or stronger; sometimes it makes your legs wobbly. In this case, regular practice may help you overcome this unfortunate side effect of panic. Remember too that a live situation may present obstacles—people, traffic, trees. Check your agility. Create a simple obstacle course—jump over something and keep running (more on this in chapter 11).

Practice running backward. You might only have to do this for one or two steps during an attack, but if you trip and fall in those crucial seconds, all your sprinting practice will be for naught. Turn your head to see what is behind you. Pay attention to your weight distribution.

Lean forward just a little. Kick backward, reaching with your legs and feet and pulling the ground toward you with the balls of your feet.

If you have young kids, practice getting away with your stroller or carrier of choice. If you use a carrier, how fast can you run safely while wearing it? Practice getting your child out of the stroller and into a carrier or vice versa. How quickly can you do it? (Never practice with your child in the stroller or carrier! More details about these skills in chapter 11)

Always run to safety, not just away from danger. This is an important distinction. Don't run blindly away from an attacker only to run into something just as bad, like an oncoming eighteen-wheeler.

> *Run to safety, not just away from danger.*
> —Michael Jerome Johnson, fight choreographer

Do Voices Carry?

A good blood-curdling scream might alert help, but I wouldn't count on it as your only strategy. There are many places where people ignore noise. In cities, car alarms, street parties, and random frenzied cursing inures people to loud sounds. Be prepared for your dire cry or loud safety whistle to go ignored.

Assuming you are trapped or being held at knifepoint, your goal is always to get away or debilitate him so he can't hurt you. A sharp scream or strategic cry for the police directly into his ear might startle your attacker and create an opening. Don't let it go to waste. When he flinches, take advantage and attack him or run. Most of us scream when we are in danger; it's out of our control. For a scream to be strategic, you must have a plan. We will discuss primary attacks and strategy in the next chapter.

If there is already a whistle in your mouth, blow it right in his ear. But if I were in danger and reaching into my bag for something, it wouldn't be a whistle. And a whistle doesn't tell people much, so if they can't see you they will likely just be annoyed.

If you don't have an escape plan, all this noise is contingent on whether anyone is around to hear it and whether that person will help.

If you're going to scream, it might also be smart to use informative words. "Help!" is vague and could make people feel like they're being dragged into your drama. "Police!" indicates that a crime is in progress and you are not a criminal or troublemaker. "I'm being attacked!" is also preferable to "Help!"

In his book, *Protecting the Gift*, Gavin de Becker advises parents to teach children to yell something specific like, "This is not my Dad!" or "I'm being kidnapped!" rather than only "Help!" so bystanders don't dismiss them as just another kid throwing a tantrum.

Recap

The positioning stage is where a criminal maneuvers you into a place or a situation. Positioning is the last opportunity to escape a potentially violent encounter by nonviolent means. Interview and positioning can sometimes blur into a single moment.

- Marc MacYoung's Five Positioning Strategies are closing, cornering (or trapping), surprise, split, and surrounding. Here we learned to look for multiple exits, watch for easy hiding spots, use our peripheral vision to track camouflaged predators, use reflective surfaces like windows and car mirrors to see behind us, and keep a weapon handy, especially in fringe areas. We learned to watch for easy hiding spots—bushes, trees, cars—and to walk down the middle of the block so as to never be within arm's reach of doorways or vehicles. We remembered to check the back seat of our car before getting in.
- We learned nonviolent disruption:
    - In the section Make Like a Tree, we discussed that the best option is always to escape but only if he won't see us, can't outrun us, or if there is a safe location within sprinting distance. To that end, we can practice sprinting against someone bigger or taller. If we have kids, we can practice (sans child) getting away with a stroller or carrier. We can practice getting our child out of the stroller and into a carrier and vice versa.
    - In the section Do Voices Carry?, we covered how a good blood-curdling scream or whistle might alert someone within earshot, only if they can and will assist us, and if we use the right words and don't only yell "Help."

Suggested Practices

 Go the Distance. If you think you're fast enough to outrun others, put it to the test. Warm up by walking or doing knee raises for a few minutes. Then practice running ten-to-thirty-second sprints with a minute or two of walking in between. Compete against a taller or faster partner for reference. Walk it off afterward to cool down. (See chapter 11 for suggestions on sprinting with strollers and carriers.)

 Hindsight. In unfamiliar territory look behind you every now and then and take in the street signs and other landmarks. It will keep you from feeling lost if you go back the same way.

Try not to look fearful. Take a picture with your phone so you look like you're doing something. Take it up high so you appear to be interested in the sky or a tall tree or building and don't upset others by taking pictures of people.

 Five by Five. Find a curious party and practice articulating Marc MacYoung's Five Interview and Five Positioning Strategies until they are clear to you. Form your own acronym or mnemonic (I failed at it), and let me know what you come up with!"

CHAPTER 9

The Self-Defense Continuum, Stage 4—Disengage the Attack

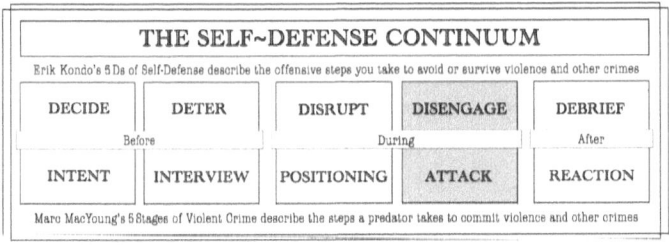

SDC Stage 4: Disengage the Attack

Things are more easily seen from the edges.
Danger rouses the sleeping mind.
It makes...things clear.

—Patrick Rothfus, *The Wise Man's Fear*

Since we can't count on the cavalry riding in or our attacker's ineptitude for our survival, we need a plan—preferably one that is tailored to us and that wasn't originally built literally for a cavalry. The best way to do this is to contemplate all available options for stopping those who are willing to cheat and who probably outclass us in strength and fight experience so we can piece together our own personal strategy.

To stop an attack once it has begun, we must learn to strategize and make radical, sometimes terrifying choices. We are about to embark on a journey into some dark territory to explore ways of surviving a violent encounter.

Someone you may or may not know has targeted you. They have come up with a plan (intent); they have evaluated you and found you to be an appropriate target (interview); they have invited you to a party, waited for you outside your office or befriended you online (positioning). Now you are at ground zero, and the attack—whatever shape it takes—is imminent.

> **TRIGGER WARNING:** This chapter may be overwhelming in places to some. Skip ahead and come back if you need to. There are no rules about how to read this book.

The Unfair Fight

> *Guard your spirit, Ketanji... for to dwell on unfairness is to be devoured by it.*
> —*Lovely One*, by Justice Ketanji Brown Jackson

What would an eight-year-old have to do to free herself from your grasp? Would her violent kicking and screaming stop you if you knew she were seriously ill and you had to get her to the doctor, or would you just grab both her little wrists with one hand, talk to her in a soft voice, and put her in the car screaming?

What if it were you against a dangerous criminal and the strength differential was more or less the same? This creates a disturbing picture of the level of difficulty you might give a calculating predator if you don't have a plan ahead of time that includes brutality, trickery, and other outrageous methods.

Strength isn't the most important factor in an unfair fight. There's height, which affords gravitational assistance, weight, which does the same and more, leverage from longer limbs, the element of surprise, and previous experience with fighting and weapons. Violent criminals often have all these things in their favor and more.

A criminal has chosen to hurt you because you have something they want and because they have perceived you to be at a disadvantage: you appear smaller, weaker, distracted, too nice; you have a baby with you or are wearing clothing or shoes you can't move in. Your assailant is fighting very dirty. So should you.

The Grand Dilemma

Options are limited at the Attack stage. Every ounce of knowledge and force you possess might not be enough. He may be bigger or stronger, he may have a weapon, he may be in the throes of a psychotic break or drug-induced euphoria, or all of the above.

You can only legally avail yourself of brutal self-defense methods under threat of death or severe injury, yet if you wait to figure out what a potential assailant's intentions are it can quickly become too late.

To maim or kill or to be maimed or killed—these are the decisions we may have to juggle under extreme duress. This is the grand dilemma: what you must do to survive versus what is legal. And you will have a minuscule amount of time to make an educated decision that impacts the rest of your life and the lives of others. The more information you have and the more consideration you have given to your traumas, training, and mindset, the better off you are likely to be when you have no time at all to think.

Deep Self-Trust

What are your belief systems? Have you ever been in dire circumstances or logged your responses to stress? Do you know what you can expect from yourself? Do you have any reason to believe you might lash out unnecessarily, or would you be more likely to freeze? Would you do what you had to and feel okay about it even when hindsight shows its long and lusty claws? Contemplating these questions in advance can fortify your decision-making apparatus. Ultimately, you want to be less likely to freeze and more likely to be proud of your choices.

When something unusual or explosive happens, you find things out about yourself you didn't know. You are suddenly filled with unfamiliar emotions—fear, anger, ego reactions. Some not-knowing is normal (we can't know how we will react to unforeseen events) but when we neglect opportunities to observe ourselves and learn from experience, we deprive ourselves of the chance to get it right the next time.

Like lots of folks, I studied taekwondo in my younger years. Never in all my years of tournament hopping, training, or teaching was there a discussion of what really happens when violence is done to harm rather than win a trophy. Years later, when I found Sayoc Kali, I was shocked by what I didn't know. Training under stress, I learned to understand what happens to the human body when it is overwhelmed by emotion: the babbling, the crying, the disturbing calm, the second-guessing, the seemingly irreversible exhaustion, the nearly paralyzing embarrassment from all of the above.

Statistically, it is more likely a woman will fail to protect herself with enough brutality than overcompensate and attack someone when she could have walked away instead. Many more women today are damaged by others than do damage. Many more women are murdered than commit murder. If you think you are likely to have trouble drawing blood in the name of protecting yourself and your loved ones, you have a different set of issues than someone whose favorite pastime is full-contact cage fighting.

I urge you to catalog your responses to different types of stress. If you are unable to trust your reactions, you may second-guess yourself when seconds count. The more you observe your own thought processes—the more questions you have answered in your head—the better you will function under pressure. Brief moments will add up to an encyclopedia of self-knowledge and allow you to trust your ability to act reflexively.

Chapter 9: The Self-Defense Continuum, Stage 4

Willing and Able

Whether you survive a violent encounter with a devious criminal may well depend on just how dirty you are *willing* to fight and just how dirty you are *able* to fight. The only way to survive a physical attack against a sociopath who is more experienced with violence than you is to use more calculation and force than you have probably ever used before.

Though many of us have hit bags, BOBs, makiwara boards, and even consenting opponents, none of it quite prepares us to feel, smell, or taste bodily fluids. Fighting, contrary to Hollywood movies, is messy. It's understandable if you haven't mulled these things over in detail. And without much data on whether considering where we stand on certain issues makes us safer and keep us from freezing, all we can do is be prepared.

In 2017, during one of the few studies on tonic immobility—also known as the human freeze response—during assault, researchers interviewed 298 women who visited the Emergency Clinic for Rape Victims in Stockholm, Sweden, within one month of their attacks. They found that 70 percent of the women reported significant freezing, and 48 percent reported an extreme state of freeze during the assault. The conclusion of the study was that a freeze response during rape is a common reaction and that it is also associated with higher instances of PTSD and severe depression.[16] It probably doesn't help that the freeze response makes it much more difficult to prove the event was nonconsensual.

I've heard quite a few women express concern that the consequences would be worse if they fight back. I know women who have been told by law enforcement that the assailant will only hurt her more if she fights back, and this has been confirmed by some law enforcement professionals I worked with. I wonder if that officer would take his own advice or give it to his wife or daughter. Aggression in men is considered manly; the same in women is often considered ugly. In some countries, almost any form of defiance by a woman is punishable by extreme measures or even execution. All of this partly explains the paralysis sometimes caused by the thought of fighting back, even in self-defense.

---

16 Anna Tiihonen Möller, Torbjörn Bäckström, Hans Peter Söndergaard, and Lotti Helström, "Identifying Risk Factors for PTSD in Women Seeking Medical Help After Rape," *PLoS ONE* 9, no. 10 (2014): e111136, p. 146, https://doi.org/10.1371/journal.pone.0111136.

Overall, an instructor's concern should be that women will fail to fight back, struggle impotently without actually fighting back, attack with minimal force, or freeze and do nothing at all rather than make a decisive attack. In the moment, the freeze response tends to last less than thirty seconds but feels longer. It may work to keep us from stepping off a cliff or to help us gather information, but during an assault we need to act, and this means we must practice identifying and breaking out of freezes when they occur.

Freezing happens to everyone. It has likely happened to you already in small ways while on stage or taking a test. The first time I remember being aware of a freeze reaction was in my early twenties. I visited my cousin while she was babysitting a friend's child. She was walking a bicycle with the child buckled into the child seat and tripped; the bicycle fell and the child with it, suspended above the ground by the plastic seat. I just stood there for what seemed an interminable time while my cousin struggled. I knew I should move, but the shock of the sudden event held me there. I snapped to action when my cousin shouted at me for help. It was a relatively minor incident and the child was fine, but the memory stuck with me. I couldn't understand why my body wouldn't respond and played the scenario over in my head for years. I've observed myself in other freezes since then and am happy to report every subsequent freeze has been shorter.

You can practice breaking out of a freeze by learning to recognize when it's happening and naming it either in your head, or even better aloud, "This is a freeze response," or something similar. Self-observation is the crucial starting point. Sometimes all it takes is recognition. Forcing movement can help break a freeze as well. Whether you wiggle a finger, swallow, or raise your eyebrows, movement puts you back in your body. If you are frozen in fear, try turning fear into anger. Fear and anger are similar in emotional tone, so it might be possible to replace one with the other and snap yourself into action. It's been said that terror paralyses, anger galvanizes.

Now it's time to fight back. Your first attack against a predator can mean the difference between his upper hand and yours. Your first contact tells him many things, including whether you are willing to fight,

Chapter 9: The Self-Defense Continuum, Stage 4

how hard you are willing to fight, how dangerous you are to him, and how much force it will take to subdue you.

You must know that when you defy a criminal, he will respond. Often, that response takes the form of a short burst of warning violence—the one quick, hard hit that does more to subdue you than a thousand words. It's sudden and devastating. Maybe you lose consciousness for a millisecond. And when you snap out of it, you're waiting for the next one.

But instead, the pain is followed by kind words delivered in a soft, measured voice, "I don't want to hurt you, just do what I say and I won't have to. Let me get you some water and a towel so you can get cleaned up. Relax, it'll be okay. I promise." (If you read *The Gift of Fear* you know the unsolicited promise is one of de Becker's pre-incident indicators.)

Violence is communication. Your violence tells him you won't go calmly while his violence says, *If you don't comply it will hurt a lot.* This intimidation technique is designed to scare you into subservience or distract you into forgetting to protect yourself, though sometimes the intention is to lead you to hit back and justify continued violence. All of this is just to say, if you have to attack him, be willing and able to give it everything you've got (more on the importance of your primary attack coming up).

There are some criminal instructions you should pay attention to and some you should not. A resource predator who wants your diamond-studded watch may tell you what he needs and, in many cases, following his instructions can keep you from getting hurt. Conversely, if a process predator, who wants to do heinous things to you in a private place far from scrutiny, tells you to do what he says and you won't be hurt, you should do everything in your power not to comply. If you are trapped or under someone's control and what they want is *not* clear, assume process predator.

You said "no" and your assailant has ignored it. He knows he outweighs you, he knows he outclasses you as a fighter, and he knows he has a gun or a knife and assumes you don't have one. He likes easy odds. Now he is forcing you into a car, onto a bed, into the bathroom; or he has already hit you as a warning to let you know you need to comply.

Don't.

A person who complies with a predator who sees her as a toy may be a dead victim, or worse. Pick your moment. Galvanize yourself. Tell him you will comply. Attack suddenly. When you do, know with every molecule of your being that he cannot possibly take you once you let the beast out. You might almost feel sorry for him, but not really—he's brought this on himself.

What if your most beloved people were with you? Your kids? Your partner? Make the raw decision now so you don't stop and question yourself when every second counts. Make a pact with yourself that you won't quit until the threat runs screaming.

Consider your ethical stance on dying and killing and the lengths you would be willing to go to in the name of survival. Could you damage someone irreparably? Poke out an eye? Could you kill someone if you felt sure they were going to kill you or your child? What you think you can do and what you can ultimately do might be very different. These are thought experiments—ways to start conversations with yourself and hack your feelings and reactions to danger so you don't freeze.

What would it take to snap you into action if you were stuck in freeze? What could you think of that would galvanize you with the mental, emotional, and physical strength to take heinous action in the name of your survival? You may need a trigger. Think about it now. Your trigger may be the thought of this guy daring to try and take you away from your children. It may be indignation and incredulity or pure rage. It could be hearing the music from *Rocky* in your head. Find your trigger and give yourself permission to do whatever it takes to survive.

If you look to the animal kingdom, you will find many instances of tiny animals outsmarting, scaring away, or fighting off larger predators with attitude and determination—the Tasmanian devil, the snake, the badger. Use every emotional and psychological tool in your arsenal to build yourself up and instill fear in your assailant. Make his resolve falter, make him second-guess his choice, take the wind out of his sails, turn the tables, and take the upper hand.

People have been shot fifteen times and stabbed over forty and gone on to live normal lives. Psychogenic shock may cause our legs to go limp when we see our own blood, but in reality the body can go on. And go on it does. Malala Yousafzai was shot point blank in the head—the rest is herstory.

Yogi Bera is right: "It ain't over 'til it's over." When it comes to violence and self-defense, your ethical systems, your dos and don'ts, your helpful and detrimental triggers and glitches are all better considered now than later.

Self-Defense Law 101

If you study or teach self-defense, you must have at least a basic understanding of the statutes and laws that affect decision-making around this complex subject. As a martial artist, you may be judged more harshly than non-martial artists; words like "black belt" or "instructor" will affect the thinking and decisions of judges and jurors.

The kind of person you are matters if want to be believed. This means, don't be someone who hurts people out of anger; don't have a criminal record; don't fill your social media pages with cracks about killing stupid people.

Following is a primer to help you make the smartest choices before, during, and after an assault. If you want more detailed information, I can't recommend any book more highly than Rory Miller's *Facing Violence*.

Look up your state statutes concerning self-defense, force justification, and weapons, and talk to local law enforcement. Know your legal rights and wrongs in the place you live and spend most of your time. What are you allowed to carry with you? What isn't allowed? Can you legally shoot the guy who broke into your house, or are you required to try and escape? Make sure your source is official. Don't take anyone's word for it, and do your own research. If you are an instructor, Miller suggests that you not only read your state statutes but understand them, print them out, and disseminate them to your students.

You've survived an attack. To literally add insult to injury, you may now have to "survive" the legal system. Here's the good news. If you only did what was necessary to protect yourself and your family, you will be fine in most cases. The clearer it is that you were fighting for your life, the simpler things are. But the injury or death of your attacker complicates things and, though you made the choice that saved you, you will be asked to explain why in detail.

What you may do legally to protect yourself is governed by this very carefully worded statement: *You may use the minimum level of force that you reasonably believe is necessary to safely resolve the situation.* Read it again. It is intentional legal jargon. What it says is that you may only injure or kill because there was no other way for you or your loved one to survive. You may not injure someone because you were angry or because they said they were going to hurt you tomorrow. Killing out of reasonable fear is defensible; killing out of anger is not. If you can walk away, you should. In some cases, you must, according to law.

Here's something you may not be aware of: if you injure or kill your attacker and it goes to court, a plea of self-defense is an affirmative defense. This means you have effectively pleaded guilty to an attack on another human being, which puts the burden of proof on you. You will be asked to prove to the people who uphold the law that what you did was necessary. If you fail to prove this beyond a reasonable doubt, you could be in trouble.

The term preclusion means you must prove that other ways of saving yourself failed or that there were reasons these other things could not be done. Taken literally, his actions must preclude any other possibilities for your survival beyond your incapacitating him.

Being in fear for your life is not enough; you must describe the conditions. For example: *I could not escape because he was holding me down and he was much heavier. I couldn't get away with my children and I couldn't leave them. He told me he was going to kill me and then he came at me.* You can use the Crime Triangle of motive, means, and opportunity as a guideline—it's likely the authorities will. Did he say he would harm you or show intent to harm you? Did he have the ability to hurt you (by being stronger or having a weapon)? Did he have the opportunity (you were alone with no one to hear or help you)?

If criminals break into your home, state laws dictate whether you can attack them or are required to try and leave. The statutes that allow you to stay in your home and fight are known by several names including Castle, No Duty to Retreat, and Stand Your Ground. The ones that

Chapter 9: The Self-Defense Continuum, Stage 4

require you to do everything to leave the premises are referred to as Duty to Retreat.

Stand Your Ground laws allow you to stay and fight, and, at least theoretically, lower the standard of preclusion—that is, if someone breaks into your home, it is assumed they have given up their rights and you are justified in using whatever force you deem necessary. Duty to Retreat means you must be able to show that you exhausted all options of escape before defending yourself with force: you were restrained, you had young kids to protect, the exit was blocked. Duty to Retreat means if you can leave, you must. If you don't, you are likely to fail preclusion and risk being charged.

Even if state law is in your favor, I strongly advise you to keep the concept of preclusion in mind. Assume you will have to justify why you had to fight if you want to stay on the right side of the law and out of prison. Among other reasons, there is ample evidence to show that Stand-Your-Ground laws do not apply equally to victims of domestic abuse, and especially to women of color.[17]

As soon as you have protected yourself and your family and assured their immediate safety, you will have to talk to the authorities. This can be very difficult under the influence of cortisol and adrenaline, which can make you feel like someone shot you up with an unknown street drug against your will. These powerful bodily chemicals come to your aid during stressful situations and temporarily shunt blood from your human brain to your lizard and monkey brains, and we know what that means. In addition, black and brown people must often deal with preconceived ideas and assumptions that they must be the troublemakers, which can cause increased anxiety and further hamper clear articulation.

I was privileged to participate in a seminar with author, instructor, and expert witness Massad Ayoob, who makes some very helpful suggestions about what to say after you have injured or killed someone in an attack on your life. Look him up and read his books. In short, he says, contrary to other advice to stay quiet or be extremely cooperative and answer every question, there is a middle ground. He suggests you make a brief statement of why you did what you did (he attacked me, I

---

[17] Zerlina Maxwell, "How Stand Your Ground Laws Failed Marissa Alexander," *Essence*, October 27, 2020, p. 153, https://www.essence.com/news/how-stand-your-ground-laws-failed-marissa-alexander/.

protected myself the only way I could), promise to cooperate after you have counsel, and point out evidence or witnesses, if you can, before they disappear.

This is, of course, all contingent on your state of mind and your ability to be clear headed under extreme duress. Police can be convincing and intimidating, and you may not have control over your mouth or your brain after you have been attacked or someone close to you has. You may go catatonic and find it difficult to speak at all. If you're unlucky, you might find you babble uncontrollably (you're running through it all in you head, but also out loud) and accidentally incriminate yourself. You might be so elated to be alive that you celebrate by proclaiming your happiness that he's dead, and announce that he deserved it anyway. And these unfortunate lapses may be recorded either by a bodycam or an officer taking notes.

> *I had the right to remain silent... but I didn't have the ability.*
> —Ron White, comedian

If all you can manage are a few words, keep it simple: "He attacked me" or "I thought I was going to die." Be a broken record if you feel you must speak and refuse to say more until you can think clearly and procure any help you need. Saying less keeps you from saying anything contradictory or inflammatory.

Now is the time to log your responses to stress and become clear about how you react when forced to discuss your actions under scrutiny or duress. If you're an instructor, learn first so you can teach your students how to respond to situations as unfamiliar and devastating as being surrounded by police after you've shot someone in self-defense.

The Three Fs (and Then Some)

You know about the three primary biological survival reactions to sudden terror: freeze, flight, fight. To them we will add posture, fawn, and submit because thinkers I respect, like Dave Grossman, have written about them, and they are relevant. Fawn could be an option to posture—a way to change the dynamic—or it could just be "a slow progression toward submission," as Rory Miller put it to me. Those with fewer options might

Chapter 9: The Self-Defense Continuum, Stage 4

fawn to appear more subservient and likely to comply. It doesn't always work, but it may cause a predator to drop his guard, which makes it a useful modern social adjunct to our built-in survival strategies.

Are these biological adaptations or social strategies? They may be both for our purposes. This is an ongoing discussion. Freeze, flight, and fight are what you did in prehistoric times against the sabertoothed tiger. And they were reasonably reliable, which is why they persist. Posture and submit are for social violence within a species. In other words, you wouldn't posture with a pack of wolves, and freeze doesn't work quite as well with other humans, but it does keep you from triggering the chase instinct in a large predator.

Let's work with these five biosocial survival reactions in the order evolution appears to prioritize them for safety: freeze, flight, posture, fawn, fight, submit.

Freeze is a common response to states of intense fear. It is what the brain often considers the first and safest course of action. The evolutionary reasons for freezing are many: to bend all our mental faculties toward information gathering—looking and listening; to prepare to flee by voiding our intestines (to lighten the load and save digestive energy); to appear inedible (the combination of stillness and extreme stink lead predators to the conclusion that we are no good to eat or that we will stay still to be finished up later, which may be partly why psychogenic shock causes some to faint); to avoid being seen by predators that hunt by movement (motion triggers the predatory chase response and fleeing is not always smart if the predator is faster). Freezing may also prevent collateral damage by keeping us from running away from one danger and into another.

We may freeze momentarily when we hear a strange noise at night. We may freeze when the guy on the street freaks out and gets in our face. Sometimes we start, or flinch first, but right after that there's a pause while our brains catch up and decide what to do (remember the OODA loop).

The signs of freeze or shock are auditory occlusion (diminished hearing) or auditory exclusion (loss of hearing) and tunnel vision (loss of peripheral vision). These responses allow your brain to shut out all sights and sounds but what your primal brain deems urgent. Unfortunately, in my personal experience these responses can sometimes be detrimental rather than helpful. Again, these responses evolved to work when we lived in caves and haven't caught up to work in modern social contexts. Evolution also favors the species and sometimes fails the individual.

With auditory issues, you may hear white noise like the sound of a rushing stream or static or nothing at all. Sometimes things will sound very far away even when they're right next to you. You may not hear your child calling to you even though you are holding her hand.

When tunnel vision strikes, your vision closes in to pinpoint the wild animal in front of you. You lose peripheral vision, which may unfortunately block the pack predators flanking you (remember MacYoung's positioning strategies of split and surrounding).

Earlier, we discussed ways to practice breaking out of a freeze: exercise awareness of freeze by recognizing instances of mini-freeze during moments like public speaking; name the freeze in your head or aloud; wiggle an eyebrow or a finger—force small movements to bring you back into your body; turn fear to anger.

After this momentary eternity, we respond based on the information we have taken in and, if possible, we flee because the body prioritizes the least potentially damaging option. Hopefully, because we've looked, listened, and smelled, we run to safety and not into the other lion waiting behind us.

Posturing and fawning are lesser-known aspects of the fight/flight survival mechanism. Posturing describes the target of an attack trying to seem bigger and more dangerous to stave off violence. In modern social contexts, this includes back talk, challenges, and physical movements like puffing the chest, putting hands on hips, and standing taller.

Fawning describes cajoling or showing subservience to appear non-threatening in the hope that the threat will feel empathy or possibly feel less of a need to assert power. It can also be used as a feint—a way to distract a predator into letting down their guard. In this sense, it may be be as much a survival reaction as a decision for self-preservation. It may happen in the moment—he's let down his guard, now I'm going to hit him with this teakettle.

Fawning is less likely to work with an asocial criminal who does not see you as human. Fawning is a common fear response and also a prey signal. People in abusive relationships may fawn, hoping to keep abuse to a minimum. It's the *if I'm nice to you, you won't hurt me* instinct. Though fawning may help in the moment, it tends to perpetuate the abuse over time since a feeling of power and superiority is sometimes the point of certain types of abuse.

The fight reaction generally comes last and is not prioritized by the brain so long as there are other options. If we are injured or killed, we can no longer procreate and so we begin with whatever our deep brains calculate in infinitesimal time to provide the best odds of survival.

To submit is to give up and hand power to the aggressor. In that sense, it could be considered a form of fawning—a hope that the violence will no longer be necessary.

Courage is not the absence of fear, but the triumph over it.
—Nelson Mandela

Fight Theory

I'm the one in class with my hand raised. I want to know why a technique doesn't feel right, why it doesn't feel like it would work for me. I want to know why, when I do the same thing as the guys, I have to perform an extra move or two to make it work for me because I'm too short or I can feel that my opponent's strength would render my response null. The extra move costs me time and gives my opponent an edge I can't afford. I want to know if there is some other technique that would work better for me. I am told to stop wasting time in class.

I've always had questions. I'm naturally curious. I need to know things. But after multiple decades of martial arts and self-defense training, I still had a lot of the same questions. I figured this was a problem.

When I became pregnant and lost my energy and muscle due to extenuating circumstances, it was a slap in the face. Now this tiny creature depended on me but also stole my strength and cognitive faculties for his personal use. Twenty years of martial arts training, and I was utterly stumped.

There are so many moving parts to self-defense, and there has been a critical lack of research invested in high-risk groups like women with young children and the disabled. In addition, so much is subjective, and there is really no way to legally, or ethically, reproduce the most dangerous aspects of being raped in an instructional setting.

This chapter is all about how to disengage from a violent attack if you are at a grave disadvantage. My quest to pick apart the insidious details of an uninvited, unfair physical fight resulted in the evolution of the Seven Rules of Disengagement. Use them as a guide to survive a brutal attack.

Seven Rules of Disengagement

Rule 1: Escape and Evade. Any option that precludes violence is a safer and smarter one. If safety is in doubt, get out. Heed all the signals of your intuition that something isn't right. Even if you fight through an attack unscathed, PTSD can have a lasting impact. Don't wait.

Rule 2: Set Your Mind. Your mind is your greatest asset and your sharpest weapon. De-escalate, problem-solve when possible, but in a dangerous encounter activate the trigger that turns you from hunted to hunter—even from socialized to sociopath. Act rather than react. Attack rather than defend. To survive catastrophic circumstances with a person bent on harming you, consider becoming the catastrophe. If you must fight, fight like you've already won.

In the wild, it's not uncommon for small animals to outsmart, scare away, or fight off large predators. Use every emotional and psychological tool in your arsenal to instill apprehension and fear in your assailant.

> *I am the weapon and weapons never weep.*
> *I'm not in danger, I'm the danger.*
> —Alejandra, Paulina, Daniela Villarreal Vélez,
> "Evolve" by The Warning (rock band)

Rule 3: Gather Information. Whenever possible, be collecting knowledge about your surroundings and your attackers. Actively listen and observe. Use the information to stay out of freeze and to strategize.

Situational awareness includes nuanced observation of important environmental elements (people and behavior, objects and obstacles, and even weather conditions), perception of the ways in which they interact, and projection of the most desirable outcome.

Rule 4: Make Panic Productive. With practice, you can learn to recognize, reappraise, and reframe your body's fear responses. Anxiety is a signal that something needs attention. Panic could be called the highest level of anxiety and indicates an immediate threat that requires an immediate response.

Recognize: By observing ourselves in lesser moments of panic and anxiety, we can learn to recognize when we are reacting rather than responding. It's partly a process of admission—the ego hates to lose control. We must become comfortable tapping our monkey on the shoulder and asking her to step aside.

Reappraise: Seeing situations and the emotions they elicit as stressful compounds our anxiety reactions. When we observe emotions without judgement, they become information rather than enemies. Listen to what your anxiety is trying to tell you, acknowledge it, even thank it for alerting you.

Reframe: To reframe is to use cognitive tools to see a situation from different angles. This may not always be possible under imminent danger, but practice is like weightlifting for the nervous system. (Caveat: These skills must be practiced ahead of time to be useful during a violent encounter.)

In a fraught verbal altercation at work, you might try to see things from the other party's reference point or seek first to understand and then to be understood as per *The 7 Habits of Highly Effective People*. If you're not finding a next step, you might ask yourself what someone you respect might do, or what you might tell someone you care about if they were in the same situation. Even substituting a less-fraught emotion like excitement to prove yourself or accomplish something difficult can help diffuse anxiety in some situations.[18] Goal-oriented thinking can help us move everything that is not helpful out of the way and focus on the most direct steps. Pick your battles, focus on your circle

---

18 Alison Wood Brooks, "Get Excited: Reappraising Pre-performance Anxiety as Excitement," *Journal of Experimental Psychology: General* 143, no. 3 (2013): 1144–58, https://doi.org/10.1037/a0035325.

of influence rather than your circle of concern, and let the excess shed away to reveal where you need to put your energy.

When in danger, the wrong questions may stick in our heads: "Why me? Why now? How could anyone do such a thing?" We might gain back some sense of control by draining the emotion from situations where people act in ways we don't understand. It might help to think of a predator as a natural disaster, a hurricane or flood, something we wouldn't have the same visceral emotional response to. There is no why; he just is. This may be helpful as a mental training exercise for mindset under duress.

When danger is imminent, panic gets you acting, listening, moving… some of the time. Other times it freezes you in your tracks. Our evolutionary survival responses are sometimes lifesaving and sometimes less so. For the most part, panic is a rush of chemicals that overwhelm the senses, the body, the mind. Even highly trained individuals succumb. The difference is that understanding and training helps shorten the length of time that you are reacting rather than responding—when the car is driving you rather than the other way around. And in the rare case of a blitz attack, where there are few-to-no indications to track, every hundredth of a second can be crucial.

De-escalate yourself with generosity. Calm your nervous system as you would a frightened child. If the internal noise is too loud, you won't be able to gather information or make decisions. To really train stress inoculation and other skills, you need a good instructor and a live class. But as always, tracking your daily responses to frustration, sudden noises, the bus that almost hits you, and that unexpected and immediate demand that you speak publicly, can help you learn to work better with your body's inherent survival systems.

Rule 5: The Best Defense Is a Good Offense. Take the initiative. Think offense not defense in a violent encounter.

This rule requires an understanding of the reactionary gap—the concept that it is faster to act than to react. The reactionary gap is a fundamental concept that centers on the relationship between time and space. Simply put, a thing that is already in motion is faster than a thing that hasn't yet begun to move.

If you cannot escape from someone who means you harm, your first

Chapter 9: The Self-Defense Continuum, Stage 4

move may be the single most important element of your life-saving offensive strategy. Sometimes our first attempt at physicality under the influence of fear is a testing blow. The urge to warn is built in—remember, we often posture before we fight; we're hoping that a show of willingness to fight will deter him. Unfortunately, if your first attack fails, you have notified him of your level of determination and his response may be to incapacitate you.

If you have decided to fight, it should be because there is no other option. If there is no other option, incapacitate him.

Make your primary attack devastating to create an opening for a merciless barrage of targeted attacks that leave him unable to recover. Subsequent attacks need to be fast and furious so he has no time to regroup, but they don't have to be quite as well planned. Commit the most vulnerable areas of the human body to memory (more on targeting in this chapter), then use the element of surprise and attack those targets with speed and ferocity.

Without a blunt or sharp weapon, or tremendous speed or power, the best striking targets are the front and sides (vascular structures) of the neck and the back of the neck (brain stem). Attack the eyes and groin only if they present themselves in the moment, as they tend to be well-guarded (more on this and other targets and techniques later in this chapter).

If your primary attack fails, it may be followed by an aggressive response. Don't give him the chance. Surprise him when you attack his most accessible and vulnerable point with your most practiced and ferocious technique and don't stop until it's safe for you to escape—whether that means he's locked in a room, tied up, knocked out, or too injured to continue. Incapacitate him and get to safety.

You can only defend yourself for so long before you're too exhausted or damaged to continue. You are unlikely to win by defending yourself alone unless he gives up or someone saves you, things you can never count on. Put him on the defensive. In a fight for your life, never defend when you can attack—in fact, attack and defend in a single move—break the action/reaction loop, and become the initiator of events. This illustrates yet another reason I prefer the term protective offense over self-defense. In a violent attack, barring outside interference or flukes the person who initiates an attack has the upper hand and is likely to continue to control events. Remember our discussion of the reactionary gap—the initiator of events has the upper hand. In the continuum of a fight, whoever attacks is more likely to keep attacking, forcing whoever defends to keep defending. I refer to this as the action/reaction loop, and you must turn it to your advantage.

The defense-attack, my clunky name for an advanced concept known in many martial arts by different names, uses an attack rather than a defensive technique for protection. Spend an evening with any number of Jackie Chan films to watch the defense-attack play out with grace and humor for the purpose of entertainment.

If an assailant lunges at you and you trip him, causing him to crash into a solid wood door, you have executed a defense-attack. Any move that accomplishes an attack and defense simultaneously qualifies. There are more elegant protective techniques than these, but in a fight for your life, always be attacking rather than defending.

Fight dirty. Use all available resources to survive. Surprise, trickery, and brutality are some of the tools you can use to break the action/reaction loop. He's chosen you because he thinks he can outsmart or overpower you. This is not a fair fight.

Surprise causes him to flinch and helps your primary attack do the job of putting you in control. Trickery is a weapon that goes way back and involves any deceitful thing you can think of. Brutality creates an opening by turning the tables on him. Brutality is usually an ugly word but not when you are fighting an unfair fight for your life. When you need it, it's a beautiful word. Brutality will keep you alive and raising your kids. Embrace it.

Attack while he's telling you how things are going to go, use a weapon he doesn't know you have—a key, a piece of hard or sharp jewelry, a plastic fork if it's all you have. Unnerve him. Scare him. Play his game, then don't. Be convincing. Appear quiet, cowed, shy, or catatonic, then explode into brutal motion. Do whatever you think will work and commit to it 100 percent.

Weapons are equalizers in an unfair fight (a primary training concept in Sayoc Kali). Learn to carry one or find them everywhere: blunt, sharp, electric, flexible, heavy, hot, slippery, stationary, projectile,

Chapter 9: The Self-Defense Continuum, Stage 4

improvised, weapons of opportunity. Always assume a weapon may be suddenly, catastrophically, and nearly invisibly introduced, whether or not you see it (also a primary training concept in Sayoc Kali). The best way to survive a weaponed attack, besides avoidance or escape, is often to have a weapon yourself (yet another primary concept in Sayoc Kali). However you feel about weapons, if you plan to learn about self-defense you must be prepared to confront them because your assailant is very likely to have one. He may not show it to you right away, but your safest assumption is that a weapon could be introduced at any point. If he has a gun, however, nothing is likely to be sufficiently protective except your own legally obtained gun (or a loaded crossbow or flame thrower), which you should be highly trained with.

Almost anything can be a weapon, so be creative. Olive oil on the floor is a weapon, or it can make you too slippery to hold on to or his hands too slippery for his weapon. A staircase could be seen as a stationary (or gravitational) weapon. Boiling water is an extremely dangerous weapon, and so is a live wire. Some of these choices can be just as dangerous to you as they are to your assailant so weigh them against the consequences of not fighting with every available resource (more on weapons later in this chapter).

Something to keep in mind: if you don't know where the safety is because you have never used it, your firearm will be of no use to you. The same goes for any weapon—you must train with the specific item you plan to use. The more weapons you train with, the more comfortable you will feel using a weapon of opportunity to protect yourself.

> *Kendra: …this is my lucky stake. I have killed many vampires with it. I call it Mr. Pointy.*
> *Buffy: You named your stake?*
> *Kendra: Yes.*
> *Buffy: Remind me to get you a stuffed animal.*
> —From *Buffy the Vampire Slayer*

Rule 6: Don't Hurt Him, Stop Him. If you can't escape, know that pain alone might not keep your attacker from continuing to harm you or your family. He must be incapacitated: trapped in the basement;

blindfolded; tied up; unable to use his arms, legs, or eyes; knocked out; or otherwise unable to continue assaulting you.

Hurting someone and stopping them are very different things. Pain is subjective. The amount of pain a criminal will be able to withstand may also correspond with his level of determination. If he is looking for an easy target, a bit of fight from you may deter him. If he is highly determined, however, and you only cause him pain, you run the risk of fueling his determination with anger. A person raised on gang violence or by abusive parents may be inured to pain. If he's hyped up on drugs, he may not even respond immediately to a broken limb.

Determination could stem from desperation, obsession, or simply an investment of time, energy, and resources. If he is highly determined, a bit of pain might only entertain him. An abusive guy who takes a woman out for an expensive meal or buys her jewelry may feel she owes him something in return. The more time, focus, or money a criminal invests in you, the harder you may need to work to avoid the full brunt of the crime.

You will have some idea of his level of commitment based on his behavior. If he won't let you leave but is ambiguous about what he wants, assume he is determined and possibly a process predator. The same goes if he tries to position you away from others either physically or emotionally. Whether a new acquaintance pushes you to leave a party and go somewhere quiet or a lover forces a move to another state, the result is that you are cut off from resources and stranded under their power. If he tries to cajole, charm, or physically move you to a more secluded place, you are likely in the presence of a predator with a plan. Knowing how hard he is willing to work to get what he wants tells you how hard you will have to work to keep him from getting it.

If you can't find another way, you may have to inflict serious damage. We are so conditioned through media to think one stab with a knife will stop someone in their tracks we often don't realize that some people can take quite a beating and keep going. Even after a person is technically dead the brain can still complete a task in progress. Even a damaged brain's final signal may be on its way to arms, legs, and trigger fingers. I say this only to bring home the gravity of the situation. If you are attacked by someone determined to harm you, you must pull out all the stops.

It ain't over 'til it's over.
—Yogi Berra

Rule 7: Never Give Up. Give yourself permission to do whatever it takes to survive, then keep going.

Deeply embedded in our social psyches are programs that deter us from acting against the rules. In *Deep Survival*, author Laurence Gonzales cites a firefighter who, lost in a national park, cold and hungry, didn't think to start a signal fire for three nights because fires weren't allowed. The social pressure on women to be kind and gentle goes deep. Anger in women is considered ugly. And most women hate to be thought of as ugly. Women are less likely to become lethal even when fighting for our lives. Fighting for our children, however, bypasses the social stigma. It is socially acceptable, even encouraged, to do heinous things to protect our kids. But fighting for your family means fighting for yourself, even when they aren't with you. If you don't have children, fight as if you do.

Kathy Jackson, firearms instructor, author, and mother of five knows that women often protect others more ferociously than we protect ourselves. Kathy begins her workshops by making eye contact with each woman individually and telling her directly and in no uncertain terms that she does not need anyone else to make her life valuable, that her life is worth protecting. Period.

You have considered your reasons for wanting to continue living and given yourself permission to do whatever is necessary for survival. In movies and on TV, people drop instantly and cease to move after one bullet or stab wound, but the truth is that much of the time it is the mind that stops us and not the body. The mind registers and reacts with shock to a first-time catastrophic situation and shuts down. As with a freeze, recognizing that you can still move and reasserting your will to live may snap you back into your decision-making brain.

Reactions vary; some see blood and collapse, others apply their own tourniquets, put the kids to bed, call a sitter, and then drive themselves to the hospital. Whoever you are, your level of commitment to survival can be critical.

In a life-or-death situation, you will need every tool at your disposal unless you want your family to endure a knock on the door from the police at 3 am. Dig for brutality and determination. Fight with everything you have. Don't stop because you see blood. If you protected yourself ferociously, it won't be yours anyway.

> *Never give up! Never surrender!*
> —*Galaxy Quest*

Weapons

Not all martial arts use weapons, but many criminals do. There are more weapons categories than you may think. As mentioned earlier, they may be blunt, sharp, electric, flexible, heavy, hot, slippery, stationary, projectile, improvised, weapons-of-opportunity, and others I may have missed. Any weapon can be dangerous to you as well, though, so be familiar with the downsides of each type.

Blunt (or hard) and sharp weapons are the best-known categories. Blunt/hard weapons break bones and damage soft tissue while sharp ones make holes in vulnerable organs or sever blood vessels, veins, and arteries. Blunt weapons are for attacking what you can mostly see on the outside: various parts of the skull, collar bones, knee caps, fingers. Think hammer, baseball bat, rock. Sharp weapons are for attacking what's inside: knife, screwdriver, a dinner fork. Keep this in mind so you don't waste your only chance on a weapon-target mismatch.

Eyes and the male groin are vulnerable to both but often well-protected. Blunt and sharp weapons sometimes come in the same package as in almost any knife or screwdriver, which means the weapon is double-ended if you need it to be.

Electrical weapons refer to anything with a charge. If you happen to be jumping your car when you are attacked, just press both ends of the cables to your attacker (though if he's touching you, you get zapped as well). I'm not a fan of stun guns, they don't drop people like they do

Chapter 9: The Self-Defense Continuum, Stage 4

in the movies, and only tend to work on criminals who are not highly motivated, but they do apply here

Flexible weapons generally take more practice to use, but a sock loaded with a rock or a metal makeup container can be an extremely useful improvised flexible weapon if you know how to use it. You are using a flexible weapon if you know how to use a bullwhip like Indiana Jones. You are using an improvised flexible weapon if you tie your attacker up with your scarf.

Heavy, hot, and slippery speak for themselves. Heavy things can be difficult to wield and don't always fall where you think they will. If you plan to use the cast-iron frying pan, make sure you can swing it quickly and accurately enough, or you'll waste your shot. If you choose to fling the boiling contents of your coffee pot, remember that liquid splatters and might burn you too—that might be your best option, but you will also have to remember to protect your eyes. If you slick the stairs with oil, remember that you may slip as well. If you slick yourself with oil so he can't grab you, you may not be able to hold onto your weapon or phone. Used intelligently, however, a paperweight, hot pan, or shampoo are all potential options in an emergency.

A **stationary weapon** is anything hard, sharp, or otherwise dangerous that you can trip or redirect your attacker into: the hot metal stove, a glass case, the hard terrazzo floor. A cliff is a stationary weapon if you push him off it, and so is a stairway.

A **projectile weapon** is anything you can throw, put in a slingshot, bow, or gun, and send flying (more on firearms later in this chapter). An electronic dart gun or taser is an electric projectile (tasers may be illegal in some jurisdictions and are occasionally lethal by way of falls and cardiac arrest; a taser in the eye may cause blindness). You could put ammonia in a squirt gun. This would be highly illegal and would rightfully be considered premeditated except under dire and unusual circumstances.

Liquid projectiles mostly disable eyes or the airway (unless you are a fireman and have a hose that will wash your attacker away while also damaging internal organs). Pepper spray is the liquid projectile you are most likely to carry as a nonlethal self-defense weapon. The active ingredient is an extract of hot peppers called oleoresin capsicum. Aimed at mid-face, pepper spray causes severe burning of the eyes, sinuses, and skin, and a hacking, reflexive cough that can last more than twenty minutes. It impairs respiration and sight and works by pain compliance. It hurts. A lot. But it may not hurt enough for him to stop, especially if he is on drugs or highly motivated. Carry pepper spray, but not as your only option. Check your current state laws (which change) and make sure you can buy and carry it legally.

There are lots of different types of sprays. Buy one with a well-designed safety release mechanism. I recommend a kubotan-type container. A kubotan is a blunt weapon around four or five inches long (both weapons are pictured below). Kubotan pepper sprays are metal cylinders with room inside for a pepper-spray insert. If he gets too close, even after you spray, you can still strike with the metal kubotan, which makes it two weapons in one, adapted to different distances.

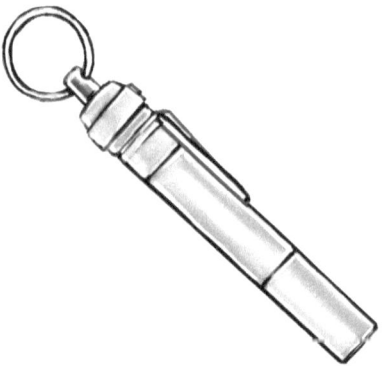

Kubotan-style pepper spray container

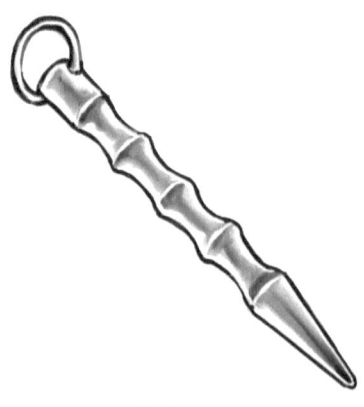

Kubotan

Chapter 9: The Self-Defense Continuum, Stage 4

Don't buy sprays that look like pens and lipstick containers unless you've checked that the safety mechanism allows you to release spray with one hand and in the right direction. Many sprays have fallible or badly designed safeties and make it just as likely you will spray yourself as your attacker. You should never look at the spray nozzle to determine how to aim, just as you wouldn't look down the barrel of a gun. Your pepper spray container should make it immediately obvious what direction you are spraying in, without looking. The kubotan styles accomplish this well.

Even the ubiquitous pepper spray requires some knowledge and practice, though few bother. If you plan to stake your life on pepper spray, go the distance. Get a refillable model along with at least one inert cartridge so you can test it. The inert saline spray exits at the same rate and distance so you know how many seconds of spray are in your container, how to aim, and how to avoid spraying from too far away. Don't forgo practice. Most sprays are only good for a few bursts. The potency diminishes after about three years, which is another good reason to have a secondary weapon. Download the detailed Pepper-Spray University PDF at ReimaginingWomensSelfDefense.com.

> If you get pepper spray or mace on you, remove contaminated clothing. It stays potent for twenty minutes or more and can easily be spread to other areas. In case of skin contact, flush with soap and water for fifteen to twenty minutes. Do not use creams or oils. In case of eye contact, flush thoroughly with water or milk for fifteen to twenty minutes. Discard contact lenses.
>
> Use of pepper spray for non-self-defense purposes is punishable by fine, imprisonment, or both. Minors, felons, and people addicted to narcotics or alcohol cannot buy pepper spray or mace. In some states, pepper spray can only be purchased from licensed firearms dealers. Mace is harder to find and less often legal.

Firearms are a loaded subject (excuse the pun) that no self-defense book would be complete without. I was not raised around guns and am no expert, but I have trained with some excellent instructors.

Read before you even think of buying a firearm: if your child encounters a gun, she should know what to do. Massad Ayoob wrote an extremely important little book about kids and guns called *Gun-Proof Your Child,* which is a play on the concept of childproofing guns, something he considers impossible. Ayoob goes through all the various ways of keeping guns out of the hands of kids and comes to some simple and elegant conclusions. It's an invaluable read for any parent.

Facing Violence by Rory Miller should be required reading for all martial artists. It also contains an indispensable section on law.

Pick up Kathy Jackson's *Cornered Cat: A Women's Guide to Concealed Carry.* Even if you disagree with her views on concealed carry and never intend to pick up a gun, an understanding of guns is a necessary part of any self-defense education. Jackson answers a lot of questions you won't find answered anywhere else—questions about things like clothing, lifestyle, and owning a gun as a mom.

Get the best training you can afford. However you feel about guns, they are out there, and it's always good to know how stuff works. If your assailant drops his gun, could you pick it up and use it, or would you be afraid to touch it? Could your assailant tell that you had no idea how to use the gun, rendering the life-saving opportunity moot? Could you tell whether your assailant knew how to use the gun or not? Could you tell whether the safety was on or off? Even if you are put off by guns (and by people who aren't), you may be empowered by learning something about them.

Whether you know it or not, your neighbors have guns. They may be hunters or sport shooters, they may have grown up around guns, or they may collect them. I have friends who are so dead set against guns they won't allow their children to own a water gun, and I have friends who take their kids to the range as soon as they are old enough.

If you have ever been held at gunpoint, it may be a while before you are ready to consider a single hour of firearms training or even some reading on the subject. Having a gun in the house may make you feel safer, or it may give you the heebie-jeebies. What we grow up with is normal and the rest is new and scary. The attitudes of the adults around us when we are children shape us. Only you know who you are and what is best for you.

Gun ownership should never be taken lightly. Bullets go through walls, and fingers pull triggers by accident. I've heard that more people are injured with their own weapons than are injured by assailants, but these statistics are hard to pin down. Gun ownership generally requires licensing, understanding of state laws, training, more training, understanding of different types of ammunition, knowledge of how to break down and clean your weapon, purchase of a specialized gun safe, and a clear understanding of how to use your gun in your house if you are invaded, especially if you have children. Oh, and more training. Your personal firearm should only ever be a danger to your assailant, never to you or your family.

Here are some recommendations for first contact with firearms:
- Start with a book or three: *Gunproof Your Child, Facing Violence, Cornered Cat: A Women's Guide to Concealed Carry*.
- Take a class. Walk into a highly rated and highly vetted, range, tell the instructor what you know, and ask which class is best for your experience level. Request a female instructor if you prefer.
- If you decide to own a gun, schedule reputable classes throughout the year on an ongoing basis with highly trained instructors. Do not count on standard NRA classes to educate you.
- Try skeet or trap shooting. It's lots of fun.
- Familiarize yourself with the gun laws in your state. Ignorance of the law will get you in big trouble. Do you know exactly how to transport your firearm to the range? Do you know if you can stop on the way to the range and go shopping with a firearm in your car? Do you know which state lines you can cross and which you can't? Don't mess around.

Improvised weapons and weapons of opportunity are similar and include anything in your surroundings that you can use to protect yourself. Specifically, improvised weapons could be described as non-weapon items that can be made into weapons, like a sharpened fence tie or a filed-down plastic toothbrush (both of which are common in prisons); weapons of opportunity would include items that are not meant to be weapons but can be used as such, like your metal water bottle or a rock.

As you move through life, try an adult version of the I Spy game and see what you can find. Classic examples are a letter opener or a broken beer bottle at the bar, but remember all the weapons categories and be creative. Almost anything blunt or sharp is likely better than your hands alone. Be realistic—you probably won't have time to pick up the copier and throw it, but you might be able to make use of smaller items to throw or stab. Sayoc Kali is where I first learned about all kinds of creative weaponry, including flexible weapons. Use a rock or padlock in your sock or your metal-buckled belt to whip-strike. I'll never forget how giddy I felt when Tuhon (Master Instructor) Tom Kier told me I could pull a pen out of the bad guy's pocket and use it against him; the idea of an assailant as my personal holster got my brain going (he also made sure to mention that we shouldn't use our cell phones to throw or strike since they serve other important survival purposes).

Practice intelligently with at least a few different items or you won't know that your pen or screwdriver can get slippery when you sweat (or if blood gets on it). Consider whether you can put your thumb over the end of an item comfortably for added power and control. Pound on a test surface to see if your chosen pen or other improvised weapon might cause you pain or break under pressure. Tactical pens are on the radar now, so you'll need to check your state laws and do your homework.

Once you've thought about how you can use readily available items for protection, you will hopefully find yourself considering how they could also be used against you. It is urgent to any self-defense regimen that you see weapons as equalizers while also being aware that they are ubiquitous and may always be suddenly, catastrophically, and nearly invisibly introduced in a violent encounter. These are more crucial concepts I learned in Sayoc Kali where all mental and physical aspects regarding the use of weapons are studied in depth.

Even a reflexive flail response to being attacked is more effective with something hard or sharp in your hand. The more items you train with, the more translatable your skills will be. Remember, the deadlier the weapon the more training will be necessary to keep it from being more dangerous to you or a bystander than to your attacker.

Basic Protective Techniques and Concepts

I'm often concerned that what passes as physical self-defense training for new students is problematic in all the ways discussed at the beginning of this book—including that it causes overconfidence without necessarily

Chapter 9: The Self-Defense Continuum, Stage 4

being effective, and that techniques are often too nuanced to be used in real-time. Less is also more; five to ten simple physical techniques thoroughly practiced across multiple scenarios may be enough for most self-defense purposes, at least early in training. Prioritize quality over quantity.

> *I fear not the man who has practiced ten thousand kicks once, but the man who has practiced one kick ten thousand times.*
> —Bruce Lee

In this section you will find what I consider best practices for instructors to teach individuals with little-to-no prior experience who want self-defense training they can utilize immediately. A book is no place to learn how to move, so I've included physical concepts, not only techniques. Along with the Seven Rules of Disengagement, these concepts apply to any number of techniques and can be used to expand a protective offense vocabulary. The techniques and targets included are ones I consider most efficient as a primary attack—the attack that serves to open an assailant up to a continued barrage. This means they adapt to multiple circumstances and have the potential to be devastating without years of practice.

If you are attacked and there is no other way out, you must be willing and able to do damage quickly. There are few techniques that accomplish this without a weapon. Kicks and strikes can be strangely unreliable. A kick that takes out one guy might not phase a smaller one. If you kick him in the gut and he's breathing in, you might leave him gasping, but if he's ready, it might have no effect at all. You might strike him and he might dodge, trip over something, and die—odd things happen when emotions are high and adrenaline steals agility and thought. It is not a popular stance that self-defense, especially the physical aspects, is in many ways guesswork. How devastating your technique is has as much to do with the other guy's state of mind, determination, experience, and random luck than with his size and strength or yours.

The idea for this book began with an urge to revamp physical self-defense. Being suddenly responsible for a tiny new person widened my view of self-defense to incorporate other aspects, but the physical stuff out there still needs to fit the women it proposes to protect. In that regard, we still have a long way to go.

Simple Multi-Purpose Primary Attack Techniques for New Students

As per Rule 5 of the Seven Rules of Disengagement. Your primary attack is your surprise attack, your first and best chance to put your assailant on the defensive, the ace up your sleeve.

A primary attack must be the easiest technique to learn in a short amount of time that stands a chance of slipping under the radar and devastating an assailant when you don't have a weapon within reach. As a practitioner learns, their favored primary attack techniques may change. But for self-defense we need to cultivate a devasting primary attack that serves the purpose of creating an opening so we can throw everything we have at him. Primary attack techniques can also be used at any time during a fight for survival, but they tend to be simple, multi-purpose, and less affected by an adrenaline dump than more nuanced techniques.

The Hammer-Fist

There is no one strike that does it all. In the movies, we see a lot of punching, but the fact is that without proper practice you are more likely to break your hand or wrist than stop an attacker with a punch. An ideal strike would be need to be simple, work from multiple positions, and do sufficient damage to your assailant without doing worse damage to the hand you may need to use to dial a phone.

One of the best multi-use strikes, in my view, is the hammer-fist. Many instructors will disagree with me. They will say the hammer-fist is not the strongest technique. They are correct. But what it lacks in power, it makes up for in other ways.

The hammer-fist uses the soft pinky-side of your fist as a pounding tool. Close your fist tightly and pound on a table—your fist is the hammerhead, your forearm the handle. That softer, pinky-side of the hand is less breakable than the knuckles (would you punch a brick wall?).

Instructors ply students with the intricacies of making a proper fist, but this applies to punching rather than the hammer-fist. The hammer-fist is forgiving—it works best when it's tight but is still effective slightly loose.

It is standard to cover the first two or three fingers of your fist with your thumb, but if you can't for any reason, you can also cap your fist with your thumb as if you've just flicked a lighter. Do not, however, tuck the thumb under your fingers.

The hammer-fist acts as several techniques rolled into one. Unlike the punch, the hammer-fist is multi-directional. Remember that you are protecting yourself against an assailant who fights dirty, and he might be behind you or at an angle, places where punching is difficult to impossible. If a man grabs you from behind, slide your hips to the side and hammer-fist him in the groin. When you practice the multiple directions of the hammer-fist, you are working toward a trained flail response and educating your body's natural fear-powered movements.

Though effective empty-handed so long as you generate sufficient power, the hammer-fist also allows you to hold a blunt or sharp weapon without any modification to the strike, making it an extremely versatile multi-directional attack.

When you walk to your car at night, hold your car key so it protrudes from the pinky side of your hammer-fist rather than between your first two knuckles (as is most often suggested) where it might tear up the delicate skin between your fingers.

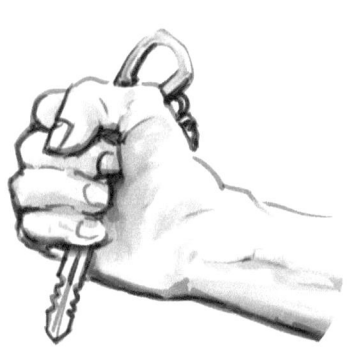
How to hold a key as a weapon

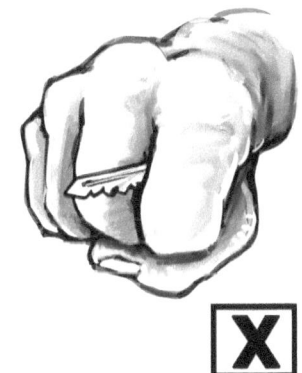
Punching with key between fingers NOT recommended

With a pencil, knife, or kubotan in your hand, you don't need nearly as much power. Almost anything hard or sharp that you can hold on to without injuring yourself will improve your odds of survival exponentially.

> You may be familiar with the **knife-hand** and **palm-heel** (pictured below), among many others. But these strikes can require more practice, leave your hand more vulnerable, and don't offer quite as many options in a self-defense encounter as the hammer-fist does.
>
>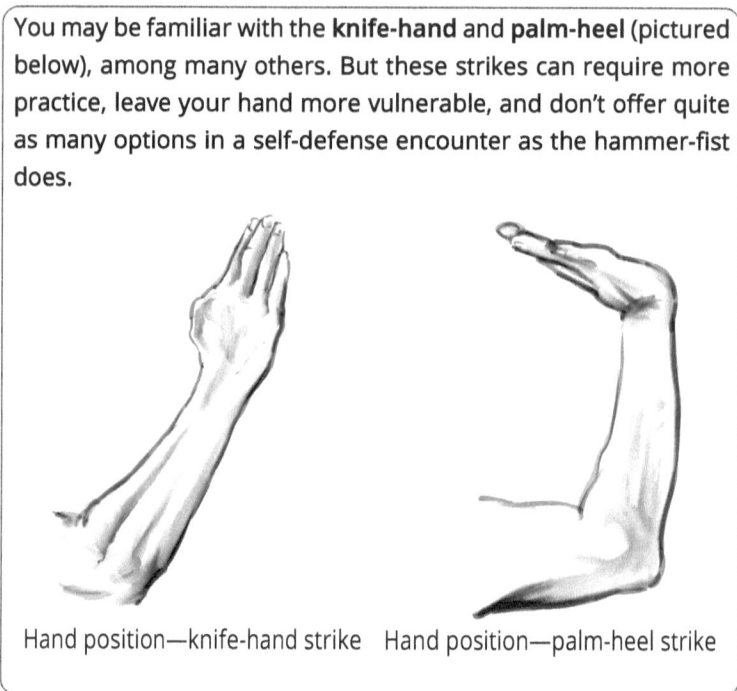
>
> Hand position—knife-hand strike   Hand position—palm-heel strike

Recommended Hammer-Fist Targets

The face and eyes are favored targets for striking, but these are some of the most protected places on the body, followed by the male groin. Here are some more available and effective targets:

- The front of the neck: just below the face is the less moveable and more vulnerable throat and trachea, which carry oxygen and blood to the brain. Crushing the trachea causes disabling gasping, coughing, eye-watering (which obscures vision), extreme pain, and even death. An attack that comes from under the chin can be hidden from the eye-line.

- The side of the neck is home to the carotid and jugular arteries, which supply blood to the brain. Temporarily occluding blood flow with a powerful strike can cause a blackout and even death. An attack that comes from the side and avoids an attacker's peripheral vision can make an excellent primary surprise attack.
- The temporomandibular joint (TMJ) where ear and jaw meet, is a known knock-out point).
- So is the back of the neck/base of the skull, where you find the brain stem. DO NOT practice attacking these targets on your partner unless she wears protection or at least covers the area with her hands or a focus pad!
- The male groin tends to be very well-defended. However, if you're on the ground crawling away and he grabs your hair, for example, you may have the element of surprise on your side, and a low blow might succeed under the radar. This is similar to the rear grab we mentioned earlier where you can slide your hips to the side and expose his groin to a reverse hammer-fist.

Attacking the groin makes it personal. It will piss him off more than other targets. Always be prepared to follow up with everything you have.

If you have a blunt weapon in your hammer-fist you have more options, including bones and joints. If you have a sharp weapon, you can pierce soft vulnerable areas beneath the skin, like vital organs and vascular areas like the popliteal fossa—the diamond-shaped area behind the knees or the brachial plexus just below the collar bone where damage can render the arm at least temporarily useless.

Hammer-Fist Tips and Training

If you haven't used a hammer-fist before, you will have to practice generating power. You don't want to anger your attacker; you want to incapacitate him, or at least cause him to freeze momentarily and allow you to continue attacking.

Practice on a heavy bag or other safe target from various angles: with your back turned away from the bag, lying on the floor, on all fours. Move your body to generate power using gravity, momentum, or torque, depending on your position (more on this shortly). If you didn't already know, pounding on stuff is a great way to build muscle without weights.

Keep your fist tight and your arm loose. Don't focus on hitting hard right away but on making contact using multiple directions and positions. Work on speed; rather than focusing on the impact, focus on rechambering the arm so you can do it again. This increases speed and keeps him from grabbing you.

The Headbutt

The headbutt is a nasty, hands-free technique that works well up close and personal when you need it most. A headbutt can knock someone out, cause great pain, or make it difficult to see through the blood from a broken nose.

Headbutts can be especially handy if someone grabs or bear-hugs you—positions you want to avoid at all costs. This usually means an assailant wants to throw you into a car or subdue you for some other reason. It helps to be on sturdy footing, but you can headbutt even if you've been lifted off your feet so long as you can wind up enough to do damage without telegraphing what you're about to do. This means practicing being discreet and using the element of surprise.

If an assailant grabs you and you are facing him with your forehead at least on a level with his mouth, headbutt him with one of the corners of your forehead—your "horns"—which are the strongest part of the front of your head (see the illustrations below). Do not headbutt him in the chin, which is hard and may do more damage to you.

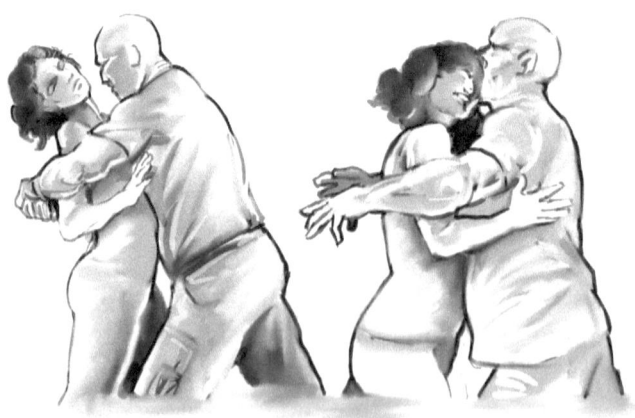

Attack to the assailant's face using a front headbutt

Chapter 9: The Self-Defense Continuum, Stage 4

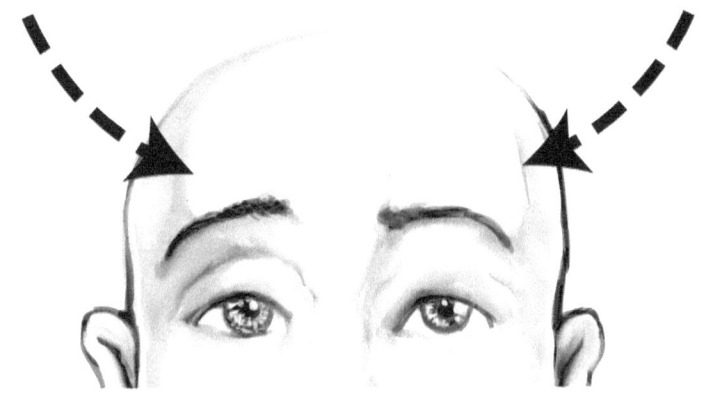

The "horns" areas of the skull

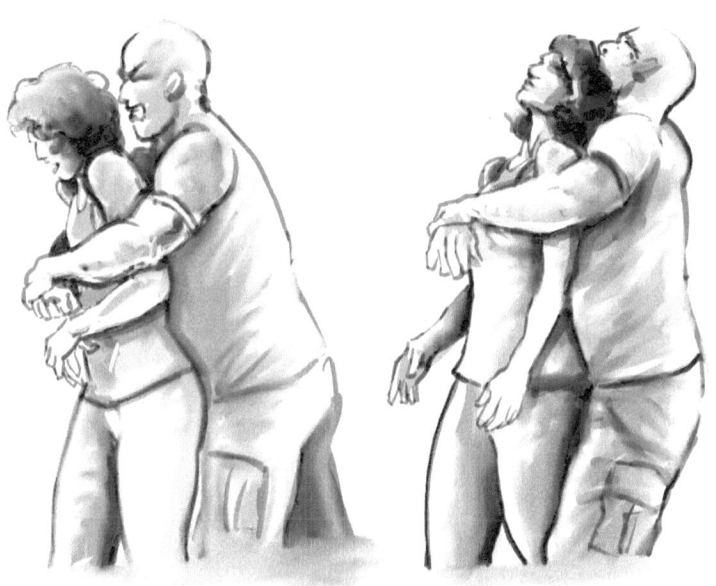

Attack to the assailant's face using a rear headbutt

If you are grabbed from behind, use any part of the back of your head (pictured above).

I'd be remiss if I didn't mention that it's possible to end up with teeth stuck in your scalp after you perform a headbutt. I don't mention this to deter you, but you should remember to get tested for certain pathogens like hepatitis if this occurs.

Recommended Headbutt Targets

- Front of the face: nose/upper lip, eye socket/cheekbones, with your "horns" or with the back of your head.
- Side of the face: jawline (where ear, jaw, and neck meet), with your "horns" or any part of the back of your head.

Headbutt Tips and Training

Headbutts are only to be practiced against padded surfaces since even minor head trauma accumulates. If you practice with a partner, use protection and go slowly. A body opponent bag (BOB) can be helpful, especially for the rear headbutt. Practice in slow motion first. Wind up sufficiently, but don't telegraph what you're about to do.

It helps to imagine an actual scenario. The first moment you recognize you are being grabbed is likely the best opening for a headbutt. Use the natural momentum of your attacker lifting you to mask your intention. As he picks you up, let your head drop to create space, then immediately slam the front or back of your head into his face. There is always the chance he will block it or avoid it somehow—there are no foolproof techniques. This is why you choose your primary attack so carefully, and also why, after your primary attack, you immediately follow up with a barrage of secondary attacks until you disable him.

Other Commonly Taught Self-Defense Techniques

Kicking and Sweeping

I'm a kicker. I began my martial-arts journey in taekwondo—a kicking art. The reason I don't focus on kicking for self-defense is that face- or neck-high kicks put you off-balance and make you vulnerable to being thrown to the ground, and there aren't many truly vulnerable areas on your attacker below the waist unless you possess an extraordinary amount of strength. Going back to an earlier story, I once kicked a five foot, six inch tall aggressor in the midbody-to-upper-leg area with my strongest, six-board-breaking side kick and succeeded only in impressing him.

Chapter 9: The Self-Defense Continuum, Stage 4

Yes, you can kick the inner knees, the knee cap, the backs of the knees, and even the ankles, but how you do this matters. If you miss the knees for the thigh, you may only give him a Charlie horse and piss him off. Remember that if he's holding onto you it may be difficult to generate power with a kick. If you are that close there are probably better options (like the headbutt, loaded hammer-fist to the groin area, or a judo throw if you know how).

I've heard instructors tell women to stomp on the top of her attacker's foot, but barefoot attackers are rare and heavy shoes or boots are standard. I've also heard the argument that a spiked heel to the top of the foot would be painful, but we're not going for pain compliance alone.

Kicking is an excellent skill to hone. Only use it as a primary attack, however, if you have complete confidence in your ability. Be sure about this.

Though kicking may not be advisable as a primary attack, it can be very useful in your secondary bombardment once he is on the defensive. There are many different kicking styles: Capoeira stylists kick while bounding up from the floor; Bagua practitioners kick with the leg loose like a whip; in muay thai and kyokushin karate, contact is often made with the shins. So long as you observe the laws of physics and biomechanics, all the different methods have something to offer. Find one that speaks to you.

If you kick in self-defense, go low and kick him below your own waist level (see the illustration below): this is where you are stronger and more balanced and where he is more vulnerable. Kicking him in the chest or belly, unless you have spikes on your shoes, is unlikely to stop him. In the interest of using your entire body, reframe a low side or back kick as a diagonal stomp. Stomping brings an emotional component that reminds us to use more than just our leg.

Sweeping is similar to kicking but with the intention of upsetting balance and can work as a primary attack if you are highly practiced. I only know three or four good sweeps, but there are many more. Some sweeps look like low kicks, some involve spinning, and some are more like scoops that pull the assailant's leg out from under him. It's worth your while to learn how to sweep. But if a kick is all you have, use it with the element of surprise. Have a plan. And once you start attacking, don't stop until he can't go on.

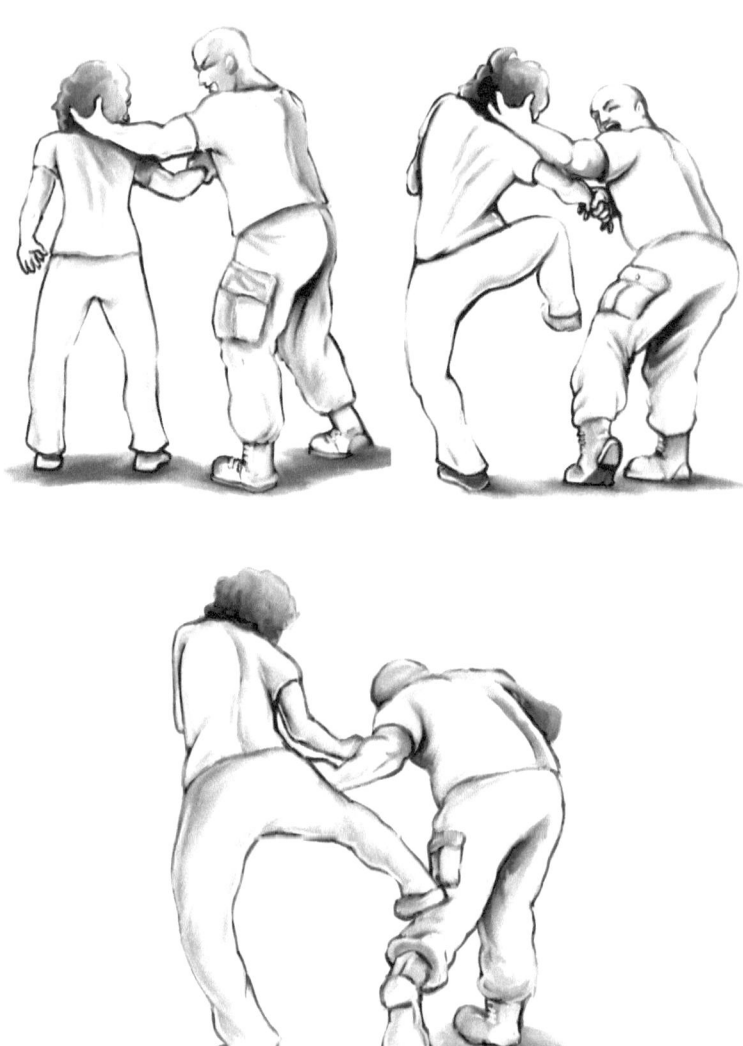

One method of kicking low (side stomp-kick)

Chapter 9: The Self-Defense Continuum, Stage 4

Elbows and Knees

Elbow and knee attacks are ubiquitous in self-defense classes but contrary to popular belief it takes a good deal of experience to generate enough power to deter a determined predator. Elbows and knees have limited target capabilities. With advanced training, elbow strikes may be useful for more advanced purposes such as getting an attacker into a stand-up joint lock.

A reverse elbow strike (an elbow strike behind you) makes it easier to generate power and can be useful if your assailant is to the side or behind you. To accomplish this you will need to properly calculate where he is based on his grab alone and without looking. If you miss and hit him in the arm or chest, you will have given away your element of surprise.

One situation in which a reverse elbow becomes more effective is if you are thrown over your assailant's shoulder (pictured below) and can bring your elbow down hard on the base of his skull.

DO NOT try this in practice unless your sparring partner wears protection or covers the area with their hands or a focus pad! Never perform this technique with full force on another person unless you are in grave danger.

The knee-to-groin technique is an iffy proposition as a primary attack since men have eyes down there and have been protecting this target since childhood. Knee strikes to your attacker's legs may go unnoticed since the femur is one of the largest bones in the body and doesn't give easily.

Again, everything you are practiced at is on the table as part of your secondary bombardment; just choose your opening and primary attack carefully.

Reimagining Women's Self-Defense

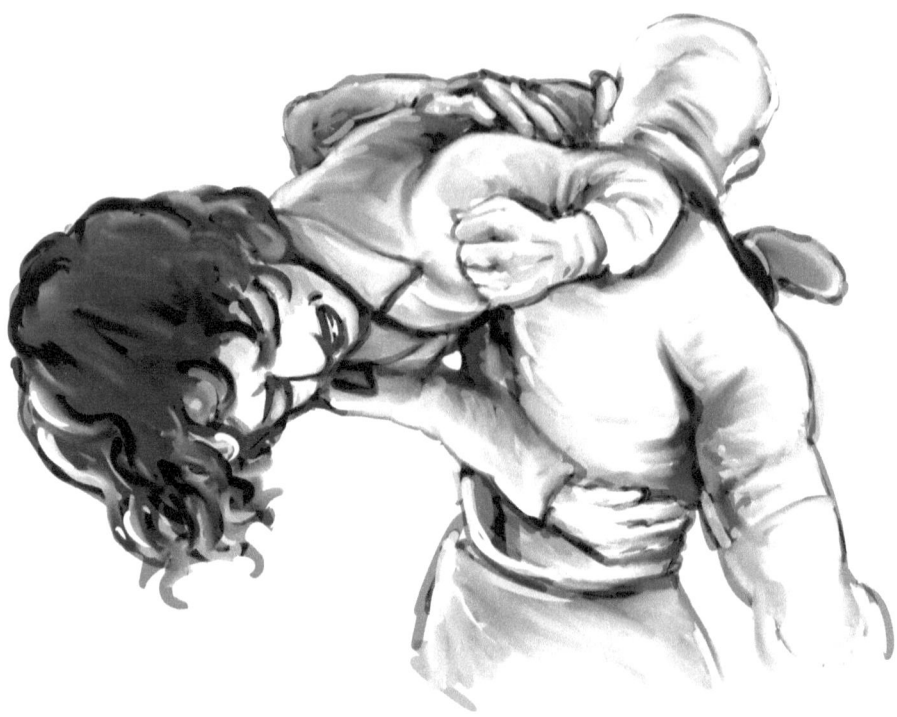

Reverse elbow strike to the base of assailant's skull

Biting and Eye Gouging

We can assume biting and eye gouging are effective techniques, though they are difficult to gather real data on. Biting and eye gouging are only for use in the most desperate of circumstances. They don't take a lot of training, but they do require a high degree of urgency and a strong stomach. The difficulty isn't in knowing how, it's in the space between thinking and doing. There is a risk with techniques this vicious: if you don't fully commit and do sufficient damage, you may incite an even more vicious response. If you are capable of fighting this dirty, he needs to make sure you don't get another chance.

Though eyes are often cited as one of the best targets, the eyes are highly protected. Therefore eye gouging is only advisable as a primary attack if you find your hands near his head already. Anchor your fingers in his hair and use your thumbs to gouge one or both eyes.

People always ask me about biting. If you feel you are about to die and you are close enough to your assailant to bite, it's an option. Biting off a finger might work, but there are many other things that aren't nearly as difficult to explain to police (though this should never be an issue if your life is truly on the line).

It's possible that biting might cause your assailant to run screaming but again it might cause a vicious backlash. If you bite into an artery, your attacker might bleed out (look up the famous jugular biting scene in the show *The Walking Dead*), but bleeding out can take longer than you might imagine, and you will have to keep fighting in the meantime. Large amounts of blood near your face could make it difficult to see.

There is always a risk of freezing with "wet" techniques like biting and eye gouging. Primal programming discourages us from doing this to another person, and primal fear of pathogens reminds us that any illness your assailant has may be his gift to you if you survive the encounter. In a life-or-death situation, contracting an illness shouldn't be a consideration, but your subconscious may register it and try to stop you.

Chokes

There are two categories of choke: blood choke and air choke. The blood choke occurs at the sides of the neck and cuts off jugular or carotid blood to the brain. Applied correctly, this takes debatably five to twenty seconds. The air choke closes the trachea or larynx, cutting off air, and takes again debatably ten to thirty seconds or more. The air choke is painful and more likely to cause submission in class, but it takes longer (as long as your assailant has oxygen in his blood) to incapacitate, and he will be fighting you while you try to hold on. The air choke is also more dangerous to practice due to the serious risk of crushing the trachea, among other things. Side-of-the-neck blood chokes are likely to require less strength and to be faster and more reliable in self-defense.

In my experience, chokes are often taught incorrectly. Unless a choke is perfectly administered or uses a lot of force, it may not work as advertised. Times vary from person to person and, depending on the precision and strength of your choke and the physiology of your assailant, a choke may incapacitate him or may not work at all. I once frustrated a guy for what seemed an interminable amount of time while he sat on me and tried to choke me with a rattan stick across my trachea using his full body weight. My neck was sore for a week, but the attack didn't come near to incapacitating me.

Explore chokes carefully. Remember that choked people fight desperately when they are starved of blood and oxygen and can do a lot of damage while you wait for them to pass out. To practice and become good at choking means you need to choke a lot of different people and be choked by them. Research on cognitive impairment (acquired brain injury or ABI) from compression of the neck, resulting in repeated transient asphyxiation, is ongoing.[19]

Joint Locks

I don't have a lot of joint lock training, and a book is no place to learn this nuanced art. Joint locking is a specialty and takes years and dedication to master, making it a less effective option to teach for immediate self-defense purposes.

The one exception might be finger locks. The small joints of the fingers are vulnerable to being bent in just the right (wrong) way, and if you find someone who can show you precisely how, these small motions can be a very useful and not terribly time or repetition-heavy addition to a self-defense arsenal. A few good lessons may be enough for you or your students to put them into practice.

If you have a more debilitating option, take it, but in a pinch, an assailant who can't grab you or hold a weapon is a less-dangerous assailant.

Bonus Technique: The Tactical or Power Slap to the Ear

I am including the tactical ear slap as a possible primary and excellent secondary attack. I have some experience with it and several people I respect hold it in very high regard. Like the headbutt, it is not a technique that can be graded for effectiveness but only be vetted by military operators, bouncers and law enforcement personnel—like

---

19 Lucas J. H. Lim, Roger C. M. Ho, and Cyrus S. H. Ho, "Dangers of Mixed Martial Arts in the Development of Chronic Traumatic Encephalopathy," *International Journal of Environmental Research and Public Health* 16, no. 2 (2019): 254, https://doi.org/10.3390/ijerph16020254.

Chapter 9: The Self-Defense Continuum, Stage 4

Marc MacYoung (a professional bouncer and street fighter), and Rory Miller (a career corrections officer and military operator)—who have multiple, firsthand experiences of varied types of violence.[20]

My main concern is performing this technique without it being blocked. However, if you succeed, slapping with the hand slightly cupped and fingers together presses air into the ear canal and can cause permanent deafness (not to be taken lightly). Proper execution also puts the base of the palm—the hardest part of the hand—at the TMJ knock-out point, making it act like two strikes in one. The effect can apparently be so devastating as to entirely disable most people. This is probably due to extreme pain and damage caused to delicate structures deep in the ear canal and to the temporomandibular joint with its associated nerves and blood vessels, which can trigger ear ringing, temporary or permanent hearing loss, and general confusion of the senses.

Ear-Slap Tips and Training

Keep your fingers together and hand slightly cupped. Aim for the center of the palm to impact the center of your assailant's ear. Think of your arm as a whip. This is a quick, explosive motion—not a wide windup. It's more of a fast flick using your hips to create power through torque. A perfect slap will put the hard base of the palm at the earlobe, which is also right over the temporomandibular joint, with the base of the cupped hand over the ear. Try different positions and trajectories. Try coming from a bit behind and over your assailant's shoulder to avoid his eyeline.

Never use any speed or force in practice against a partner. The best practice partner for this technique is a body opponent bag (BOB).

The double ear slap is also devastating but less powerful, easier for your assailant to stop, and requires both of your hands to be free.

The arm movements of the slap and hammer-fist are similar enough that training either one will strengthen the other at least within the same trajectory.

---

20 The experience of violence professionals may not speak directly to women's self-defense but can still supply some important clues, since it is difficult or impossible to compile and confirm data on the efficacy of specific techniques from single-person experiences involving trauma.

Concepts

On Being Grabbed or Held, Stand-Up Grappling, and Ground Fighting

Use all the skills outlined in this book to maintain distance and avoid being grabbed or held, which puts you at a potentially fatal disadvantage against anyone who outweighs you or is in possession of a weapon, which, as I've said before, you should always assume could be brought into play. My experience with grappling is limited, but here's what I have gleaned in my travels.

Judo, jujitsu (Japanese), and Brazilian jiu-jitsu (BJJ) are some of the arts best known for teaching students to control an assailant's body while standing or on the ground, but there are others. Look for a creative teacher who is open to your questions about quick ends to dangerous situations rather than competition. Many styles spend what I consider to be excessive time on techniques built for matched-weight training sessions or competition (one person submitting another in the presence of very specific rules).

Get extremely comfortable with a few debilitating attacks you can execute from multiple positions on the ground. Practice them ad nauseum. Ronda Rousey, an important and talented judo, MMA, and UFC stylist, made a career of a single arm bar. This isn't to say she wasn't skilled in many aspects of fighting, but her personalized armbar won the vast majority of her UFC fights. A dislocated shoulder and elbow can make your attacker less dangerous. These techniques require time to learn and the guidance of a talented instructor.

If you are grabbed by an arm or both arms, don't fixate and forget you have legs and a head to fight with. If you are grabbed by one wrist, or even both, do not fixate on that either. Don't waste valuable time trying to escape his grasp and forget the rest of your body. Your attacker may be fixating as well, which means he is vulnerable to a surprise attack somewhere else. You need him to let you go, especially if he's trying to move you to a secondary location, like to a car or somewhere his accomplices await. In most cases, he will expect you to try and shake loose, pry him off, or at least pull away. Surprise him by moving explosively toward him and using your free arm or your head to attack him with

Chapter 9: The Self-Defense Continuum, Stage 4

your hammer-fist or headbutt. You might even pull away for a second, as he expects, and then, when he drags you back toward him, launch into him using his own power against him. Now he's on the defensive, and you are bombarding him relentlessly until he runs or is debilitated.

On Footwork

There are countless footwork patterns across martial arts. In many styles, footwork is very specific, but in a fight what you want is balance and agility, and the fastest way to achieve them is often to use what you already know and hone it. If you have missed out on footwork, or you are looking for a solid starting point for your students, boxing offers a simple, effective footwork style that is easy enough to access in person or online. Anyone who dances has a head start and can adapt those skills.

Practice pivoting, catching balance, and stepping or jumping over obstacles. Connect to your core and become agile and light on your feet. Your core stabilizes the bulk of your weight so your legs are free to move. It is primarily the core that causes jumpers in all sports to appear to hover in midair.

Practice proper walking technique. Shoes (especially crummy ones) and asphalt have changed the way we walk and caused us to use our legs as stilts rather than springs. We were not built to walk heel-toe. Straight legs inhibit speed and agility. Many chronic hip, knee, and even ankle issues can probably be traced to heel-walking. When the heel hits the ground first at the end of a straightened leg, it sends shockwaves through the knees, hips, and even lower back, imposing constant wear and tear on those structures. When you soften your knees as you walk and lean slightly forward (almost as if falling forward), the balls or flats of your feet reach the ground first rather than your heels. Walking this way uses your hips, knees, and ankles as springs, allowing for quicker movement in a pinch with a greatly reduced chance of both chronic and ballistic injury.

On Falling

Falling is an area of self-defense training that shouldn't be ignored. Attacks on women often involve being grabbed, pushed, pulled, or thrown to the ground. Panic, chaos, and obstacles also cause people to fall. Falling on concrete can cause serious injury and keeps you from fighting or escaping. The average person is more vulnerable on the ground than on their feet.

Learn multiple ways of falling. Different arts advocate different methods. Techniques for falling to the front and side on a hard surface are more elusive and complicated. Many arts advocate a forward shoulder roll if you are pushed from behind, but this requires hundreds of repetitions to master and is ill-advised on concrete. It also requires youthful and resilient bones.

It could also be seen as naïve (if not dangerous) to imagine you will be able to manage a roll when you are unexpectedly pushed. The most you can hope for if you can't stay on your feet is to convert any forward or side fall into a backward fall, if at all possible. If you fall forward and don't have time to get up, you might roll to face upward. Once someone has pinned you face down on the ground, it is much harder to regain your feet or fight back.

To practice a backward fall, separate your feet shoulder width or more and protect your face and head with your hands and forearms; bend your knees and perform a deep squat, put your butt on the ground (careful of your coccyx bone at the very tip of your spine), and roll backward with your head tucked forward to keep it from hitting the ground. (The whole sequence is pictured below.) Try any practice fall in slow motion, the first few times at least, to safely build muscle memory, control, and strength.

Try to see the series of pictures as one fluid, nonstop falling motion. As illustrated below, as soon as you are on the ground, roll immediately onto your side, continuing to turn fluidly into a standing position. Notice that as soon as you turn to the side on the ground, your feet should be up to allow you to kick at his ankles or knees to keep him away, cause him to fall, or keep him from climbing on you.

Chapter 9: The Self-Defense Continuum, Stage 4

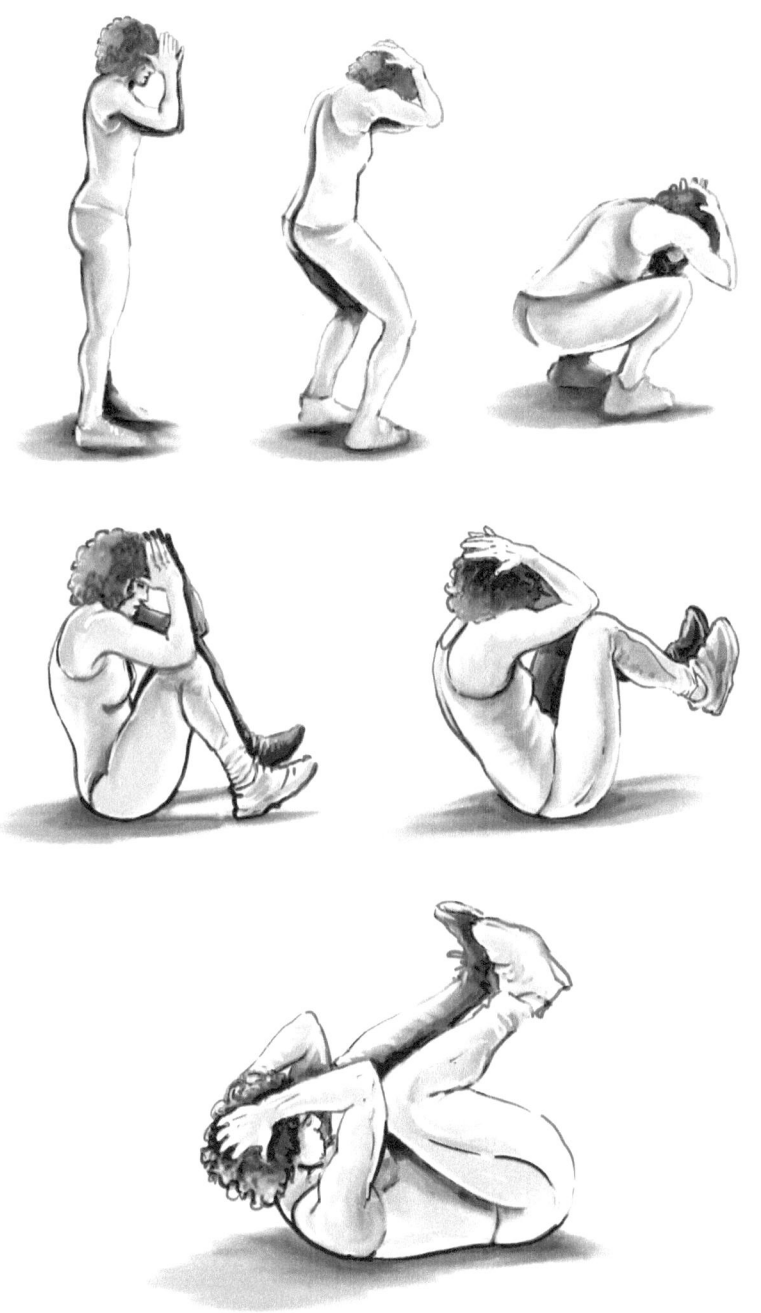

Backward falling sequence

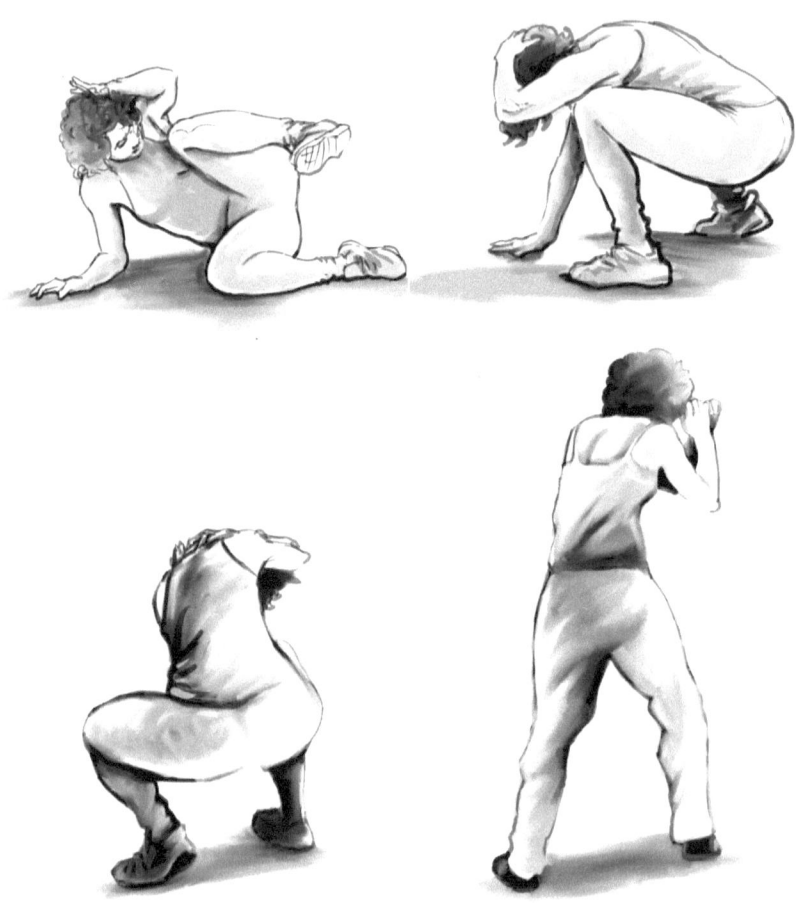

Backward falling sequence (continued): return to standing

I like this method because keeping your hands up protects your head as you roll. The turning and twisting motion allows you to watch your surroundings, creates a moving target, and gives you directional options for running or confronting multiple attackers on the way up from the ground.

Some arts perform a kind of curtsey on the way to the floor, which may be helpful if you are moving or walking when you fall and you can't get your feet into a squat position. As illustrated below, to try falling this way, place one leg behind you in a curtsey, roll across the outside of your lower leg (to keep your knee from hitting the ground), and sit on the ground. Use your leg(s) to maintain distance and fight him off if you need to. The rest is the same as the first method—roll immediately onto your side, continuing to turn fluidly into a standing position.

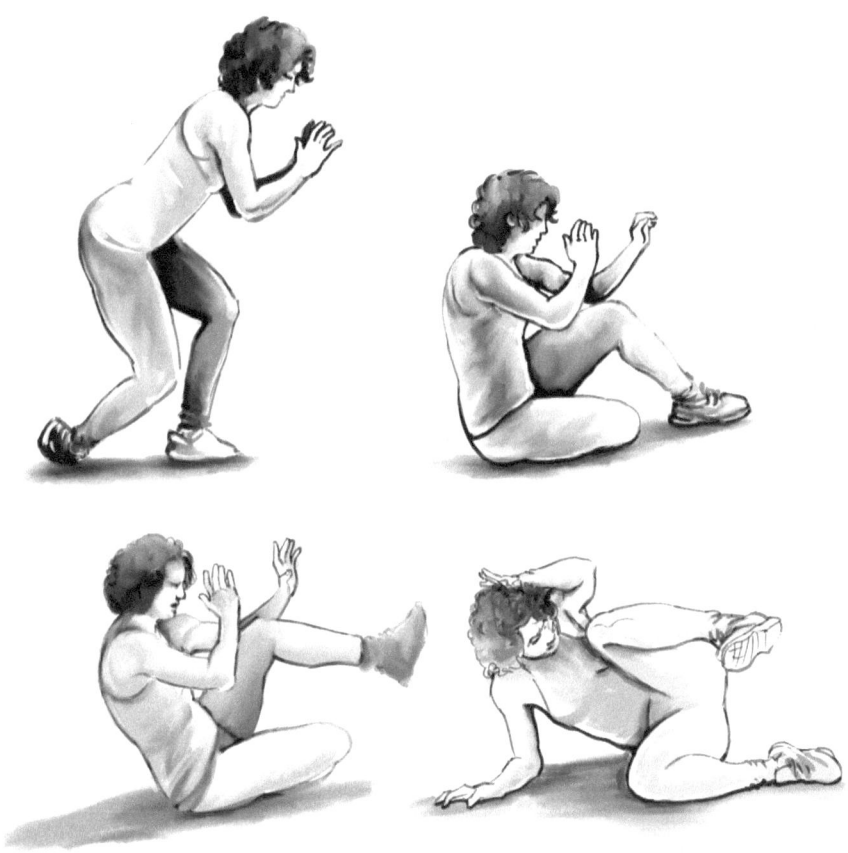

Curtsy falling sequence

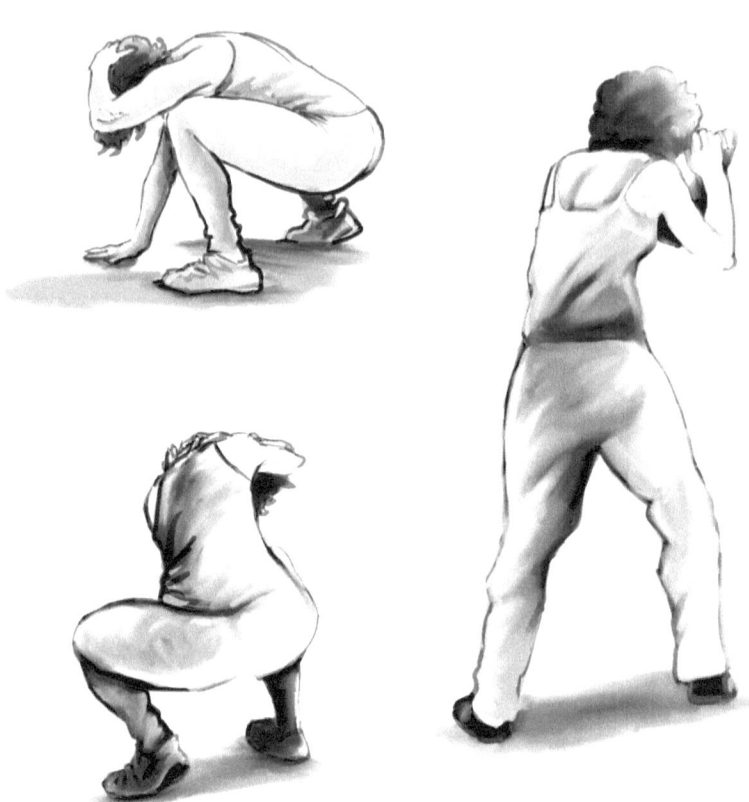

Curtsy falling sequence (continued): return to standing

Practice both the squatting and curtsey methods so you have options whether you are standing still or moving.

Another method of landing involves slapping the ground with outstretched arms mid-way between your shoulders and hips. This is common in many styles. It dissipates force across a larger surface area and cuts down on joint shock.

Chapter 9: The Self-Defense Continuum, Stage 4

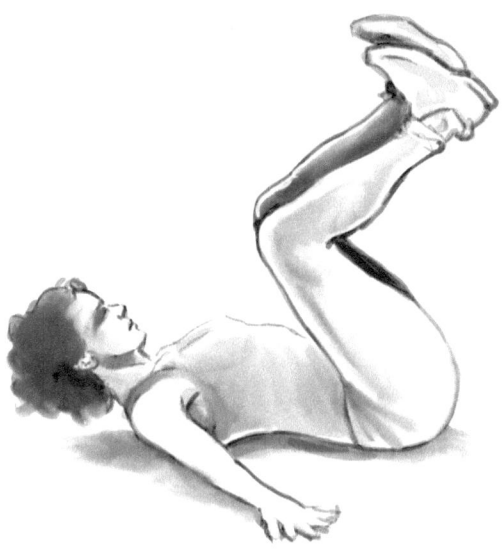

Popular alternate way of landing on the ground from a fall

I don't recommend this method of falling in self-defense since you don't know what might be around you (glass shards), and you will need your arms to protect your head and vital organs even while falling. Though I have found it useful to dissipate the force of falling in non-self-defense situations, and often flailing out is reflexive, you will have to be the judge of what is best for you. If you are holding a child, you won't have this option anyway.

If you begin to fall or, God forbid, are forced to fight with a baby in your arms, immediately pull her head to the crook between your neck and shoulder. It makes protecting her head reflexive when it is close to yours. This is a tall order since you may not have any notice. The best I can offer is to consider this position if you must run from someone, so the baby is already in position if you fall. A larger child makes things more complicated. Velcro, a simple game to help you teach small children who can't walk or run to hang on to you, can be found in chapter 11.

Reimagining Women's Self-Defense

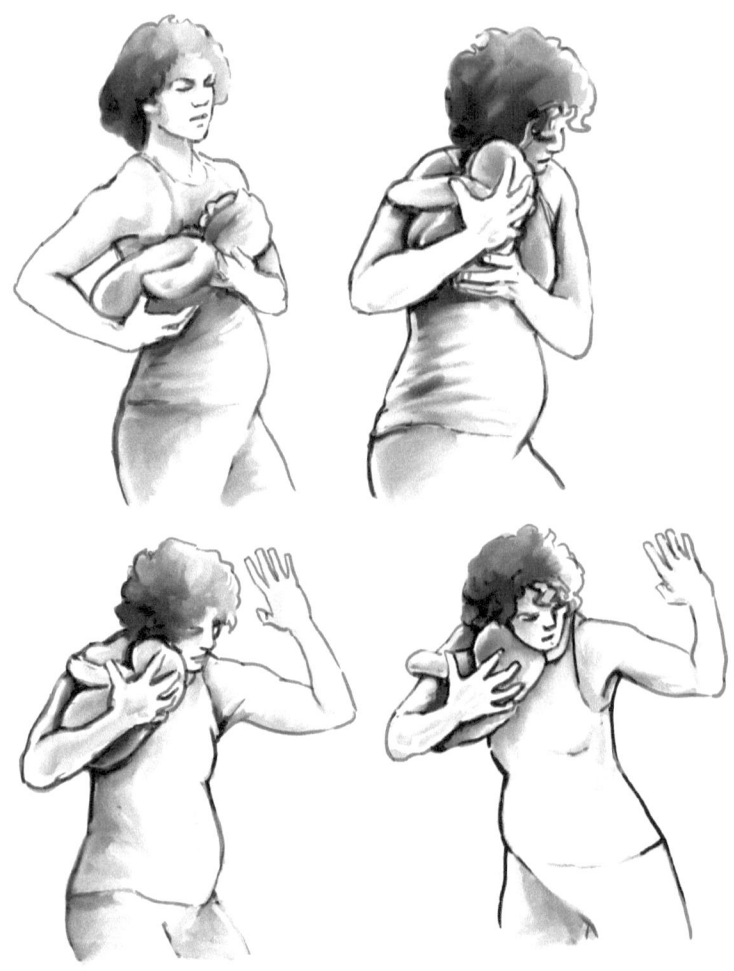

Preparing to fight or fall while holding baby

Clearly, there is no ideal way to fall on a hard surface. But thoughtful methodical practice might save you grave injury. Always practice falling on a padded surface in slow motion. This helps create muscle memory and works all muscles involved.

Don't forget to practice getting up and down from multiple positions while protecting your head. It's good exercise and will come in handy if you find yourself on the ground and scrambling to get up, get away, or fight for survival.

Chapter 9: The Self-Defense Continuum, Stage 4

Many arts practice falling and moving on the floor. Brazilian jiu-jitsu reverses what most arts do and spends 90 percent of its time on the ground. In this case, be sure to allot ample time to remaining standing or getting up offensively. In some schools of krav maga, ground techniques are focused on doing only the amount of damage necessary to allow you to get up again. I agree, as the greater weight of an attacker can make the ground a dangerous place for anyone who lacks extensive ground-fighting experience. As soon as your assailant pins you, he will do whatever it takes to keep you from fighting. This affords you minimal time to turn the tables.

I recommend exploring at least two kicks, strikes, chokes, joint breaks, and positioning maneuvers while on the ground. Use scenarios to keep things real. Plenty of people will disagree with my assertions. Practicing and discussing your thoughts with fellow martial artists are the best ways to understand subtleties and come to your own conclusions.

Basics of Power Generation: Grounding (or Rooting), Coiling, and Center of Gravity

Four ounces deflects a thousand pounds.
—Core principle of tai chi

Most martial arts and sports utilize concepts of power generation, but I rarely hear them articulated fully. There are other elements, but grounding, coiling, and center of gravity provide a strong framework to build on. These are internal concepts, and often training does not go deep enough to fully explore them.

Grounding is a feeling or sensation that leads to power generation. It describes the process of softening lower joints, sinking body weight, and spreading the feet to grip the ground. In movement, grounding uses intermittent contact with the ground for balance and a stable platform from which to gather power. In internal arts, grounding is often called rooting, a useful analogy that describes what the practice feels like.

Coiling describes the creation of torque or rotational force. It is the difference between hitting with a single limb and hitting with your entire body. Learning to swing a baseball bat is one simple way to understand this concept. If you just swing with your arms, it will be hard to hit a home run. Watch a major-league batter and you will see the building of power from the ground up into a whip-like motion involving the entire body and ending in accumulated speed and power at the tip of the bat as it connects to the ball.

Without coiling, you risk using only the brute force available to you by way of weight and strength. Coiling increases power generation geometrically and enhances just about every self-defense technique.

Center of gravity (COG) is as much a feeling as a place on your body. Theoretically, it's located where a body's weight is balanced in reference to gravity, but human bodies move, which means the center of gravity moves. In thought and training, at least with both feet on the floor, COG tends to reside somewhere behind the belly button, toward center mass, or lower toward the pelvis.

Wrapped around your COG, in a way, are your core muscles, which include the abdominals, obliques, erectors, diaphragm, and pelvic floor muscles, among others. Core strength allows you to feel and control your center of gravity and to "reach" out with your limbs while maintaining unity and stability. The core and COG create a kind of hub or central station where power can be gathered from moving muscles and limbs and directed to others.

Power generation is the synergistic process of gathering strength from the entire body using grounding, coiling, and center of gravity, among other things. Of course, all this happens fluidly in the body rather than the mind. By connecting to the ground (grounding or rooting), gathering power at your center (COG), and spiraling body mechanics (coiling), we can aspire to a key principle of tai chi (often spelled taiji) which says, "Four ounces deflects a thousand pounds."

> *It takes guts to train your internal environment. The first few steps are often a battle with the ego.*
> —Albis Suarez, strength and movement coach

Chapter 9: The Self-Defense Continuum, Stage 4

> Some of the people who are best at generating and focusing power into one target practice internal martial arts like tai chi (taijiquan), bagua (baguazhang), and hsing-i chuan (or xingyi), also known as the three sisters of the Chinese martial arts. These arts take many years to cultivate and are not generally recommended for immediate self-defense purposes. They are excellent for physical and mental health, however, and will geometrically boost any self-defense training you engage in. You may also find some of these principles in systema, where it's possible they will be more immediately accessible for protecting yourself.

Final Note on the Primary Attack

An effective primary attack is a devastating surprise attack that creates an opening for you to bombard your assailant with subsequent attacks. Your primary attack is your most well-thought-out and well-practiced technique. You may only have one chance to create an opening before he is alerted to the fact that you are a fighter.

After your primary attack, follow up with your most practiced and debilitating options. If necessary, claw and bite. But you'd better not be squeamish about blood in your mouth or under your nails. You may not know these things about yourself until the moment your survival is in question, but they deserve consideration. If he's less determined or afraid of disease, being bitten might cause him to release you; if not, he is likely to respond even more harshly. These are thought exercises, not dark mindsets to live in.

The hammer-fist and headbutt are simple primary attacks that can be practiced and used in self-defense without years of training. Try the loaded hammer-fist from medium range and the headbutt from close range. There aren't many self-defense techniques as simple and immediately useful that I recommend without extensive practice. Other techniques I mentioned, like sweeps and judo throws, make excellent primary attacks but require more time and training.

Train Intelligently—
Seven Training Tips of Protective Offense

The way you train matters. Here are some suggestions to make your ongoing training relevant and effective for self-defense purposes.

1. **Observe the Rule of Equal Motion:** Practice each technique with the assumption that you have the same time-to-movement ratio as your potential attacker. Never assume you can move faster than an unknown opponent.

I practiced taekwondo as a teenager, dutifully posing while my partner performed multiple blocks, kicks, and takedowns and allowed me to do the same. In demonstration, this looks impressive, in reality, it's deadly. My male cohorts were mostly focused on competition while I was concerned about more urgent self-defense issues.

The concept of equal motion tells us never to fool ourselves into thinking or practicing as if we are faster than an unknown attacker. We are working toward mastery of an event of which we possess no prior knowledge. Since we don't know the parameters of a potential attack, we must work under the assumption that all players move at the same speed—we must remind ourselves to factor in a reasonable yet theoretical block of time for each attack and response. This calls on us to play both roles in our minds and to assume both participants are fighting with equal urgency. If you expect to be moving constantly in the name of survival, expect the other guy to do the same. Regardless of skill or motive, he is unlikely to stand still while you practice gymnastics. Newton's Third Law says for every action there is an equal and opposite reaction. Expect a response to everything you do.

2. **Repurpose Pretrained Neuromuscular Pathways** (RPNP): If you plan to rely on a technique for survival, it must be embedded in your muscle memory and accessible without conscious thought. To this end, you can perform ten-thousand repetitions of a technique or you can match it to familiar movement patterns that you use every day. In Sayoc Kali this key learning multiplier is known as Holistic Mind training.

You can use the RPNP method by matching any new or old protective techniques to a familiar daily task or movement; think of a knee strike as climbing stairs, a reverse elbow strike to someone behind you

Chapter 9: The Self-Defense Continuum, Stage 4

as pulling open a heavy door, or an open-handed face-block with an upward elbow strike as smoothing your hair. These familiar movements can be relied on even when you are not at your best because they are already part of your physical vocabulary.

Matching old and new protective techniques with common daily movements will help to embed techniques in the body. As martial artists we know that when movement lives in the body, bypassing the slow, logical brain, techniques become more reflexive and instinctive; they may need to be tweaked for power generation and balance, but beginning with familiar preset patterns greatly speeds the learning process. Less forethought equals faster reaction time and more reliability.

3. **KISS—Keep It Simple, Sister:** Make the fighting techniques you plan to rely on simple and automatic.

When I ran Art of War, a martial-arts performance troupe that created spectacles for movie premiers and product releases, I worked with some of the physical geniuses who were capable of the spectacular acrobatic fight displays we see in action movies. When my son was younger and we watched these movies together, he would ask me, "Would that work in a real fight?" I hated to disappoint him but had to answer that Hollywood stunt fighting was about as relevant to self-defense as dance. I affectionately call these acrobatic martial arts displays finesse techniques because of the complexity of the movements involved. It's possible that the people who practice these techniques thousands of times until they can do them asleep might be able to use them for protection, but there are certainly faster, less risky, and less energy-consuming options in a true self-defense encounter. Economy of movement is key when every second matters and a rush of adrenaline has stolen your complex motor skills.

Where simple is better, less can also be more. For self-defense purposes a few simple, well-chosen, well-practiced techniques and concepts may serve you better than a large variety.

4. **Train Your Flinch and Flail:** The flinch response is a lesser biological survival reaction that can help or hinder. A flinch can protect your eyes from shattered glass, but if you flinch in an attack rather than fighting back, you risk becoming stuck in the role of defender. The flail describes natural protective movements prior to conscious thought—that "holy shit," hands-whipping-out motion that occurs when we're startled.

You choose the move you want to train to reflex: throwing both hands up over your head, elbows aimed forward for first contact is one possibility, dropping six inches to take yourself off-line of an attack while twisting to scan your surroundings is another. Rory Miller's Dracula's Cape could work as a trained flail.

The question is can we really train these mostly subconscious reflexive reactions; some instructors say no, some say yes. I believe at the height of my training I was able to affect my flinch/flail, and I know others who seem to have as well. It's certainly worth exploring since the benefits are obvious, but you may need to find an instructor who knows how to train these types of complex and nuanced skills.

5. **Prepare for Accomplices:** Predators hunt in packs. At no time is it more urgent to snap into ready mode than when you are confronted by multiple attackers as in Marc MacYoung's surrounding strategy from chapter 8. Once you are surrounded, the only way out may be through. Practice multiple methods of escaping or fighting your way out of a circle or group of attackers.

- Consider a martial arts and sports concept called shooting-the-gap. Find the weakest link in the group, perhaps between two distracted assailants who are talking, arguing, or unsure of their involvement, or between the two smallest or weakest. Without notice, shoot—run explosively—through this weak point and keep running until you are safe. If speed is not your forte, this may not be your best option.

  One technique that might function for this purpose is Rory Miller's "Dracula's Cape." This involves protecting your face with the crook of your elbow so your elbow is pointed at the gap you are running through. Your elbow protects your face and provides a hard "weapon" to help you punch through. Peek just over the crook or under your elbow to see ahead and to the sides. You can protect your mid-body with your other arm by wrapping it around your body or pointing the elbow to the side or back where it also serves as a secondary weapon. Hopefully, you have a blunt or sharp weapon—or even two—and can retrieve them in time. If so, use them from the same position to "tear" through the gap. This might be hard to envision, but imagine how you would walk through spiderwebs or heavy brush, scissoring your hands.

Chapter 9: The Self-Defense Continuum, Stage 4

- You could also theoretically spin through the gap in this or another position to make you more difficult to grab. Again, this depends on the situation and on your ability to both attack and protect your vital parts while spinning.
- If you aren't fast and spinning, or Shooting the Gap isn't for you, doing sudden damage to at least one of your attackers might convince the rest that you're too high risk. You'll need to be quick and brutal to take the gang by surprise and devastate the weakest link or closest body to you. Choose your strongest, most practiced primary attack and commit fully. Follow up brutally, but others may jump in, try to use your peripheral vision to track and avoid multiple accomplices, and run to safety at the earliest possible moment.

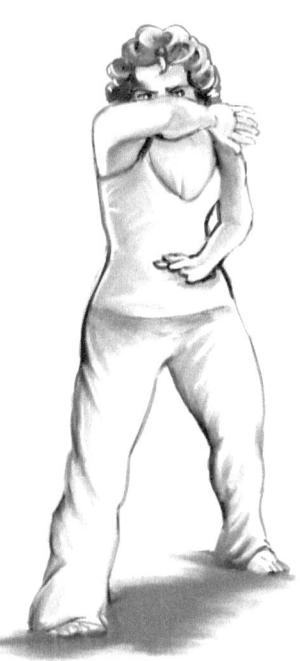

Dracula's Cape

- Practice fighting on an angle. Stay to your attacker's side and avoid the center of his body where he is strongest and can most easily grab or harm you. Try not to face him head on. Lateral and rear targets—side of the neck, base of the skull, kidneys, even the back and side of the knee—are less protected and more vulnerable than those on the front of the body. Both the center of the circle and the center of the body are dangerous places to be. Avoid them.

6. **Modify Your Training:** If you only train under ideal circumstances, you will only be able to protect yourself under ideal circumstances. Sayoc Kali is where I first learned about the importance of training modifiers—additions, subtractions, or changes to the circumstances of training that cause distraction and discomfort. Train when you are too cold or too hot; train in low-or-no light, on gravel, or an incline; train

hungry, or right after eating; train on slippery surfaces or under the influence of sleep deprivation. Safety is an urgent concern when you modify your training in this way, so take precautions.

A key aspect of protective offense is the ability to embrace discomfort. Discomfort is good for the body and the soul; it keeps you adapting, staves of mental and physical laziness, helps you appreciate the good things, and will make you a more effective more effective martial-arts instructor—and human.

7. **Slow Practice Makes Perfect:** Performing movements and techniques in slow motion prepares joints and connective tissue and guards against injury. Slow work builds strength, control and focus, and also slows time so you learn to see in between the seconds, a self-defense superpower.

Train your kicks, strikes, footwork and especially level-drops (like ducking or falling) this way. You can even practice your drills with others in slow motion. Train improvisationally by having someone launch a super-slow attack while you look for openings and launch your own slow-motion counterattack.

Recap

- The Unfair Fight: Your assailant is fighting dirty, so should you. Height, weight, leverage, previous experience, weapons, and surprise are all factors in an unfair fight.
- The Grand Dilemma: You can only legally avail yourself of brutal self-defense methods under threat of death or severe injury, yet if you wait to figure out what a potential assailant's intentions are, it can quickly become too late.
- Deep Self-Trust: What are your belief systems? Have you logged your responses to stress? Do you have any reason to believe you might lash out unnecessarily? If you are unable to trust your reactions, you may second-guess yourself when seconds count.
- Willing and Able: Whether you survive a violent encounter may depend on how dirty you are willing and able to fight. The only way to survive a physical attack against a sociopath who is more experienced with violence is to use more calculation and force than you have ever used before.

Chapter 9: The Self-Defense Continuum, Stage 4

- o Your violence tells him you won't go calmly, while his violence says, *if you don't comply it will hurt a lot*. Your first contact tells him how hard you are willing to fight, how dangerous you are to him, and how much force it will take to subdue you.
- o If you are trapped or under the control of someone whose desire is not clear, always assume process predator.
- o Consider the lengths you would be willing to go to in the name of survival. Find a trigger. Give yourself permission now to do whatever it takes to survive.

- Self-Defense Law 101: Be familiar with your state laws concerning weapons and violence. Make sure your source is official. For more details, see Rory Miller's *Facing Violence*, chapter 1: Legal and Ethical.

  - o *You may use the minimum level of force that you reasonably believe is necessary to safely resolve the situation.* Killing out of fear is defensible; killing out of anger is not.
  - o The concept of preclusion says you must prove that other ways of saving yourself failed or show there were reasons you could not escape. Keep this in mind and plan to justify why you had to fight.
  - o Castle, Stand Your Ground, and No Duty to Retreat laws allow you to stay in your home and fight in the event of a break in. Duty to Retreat laws require you to leave if you can.
  - o Under the influence of cortisol and adrenaline you may babble and say incriminating things. Prepare a mantra with only the most important facts. Try to speak as little as possible until you have an expert of some sort to guide you.

- Freeze, flight, posture, fawn, fight, submit: These are the biosocial ways our bodies react to panic. You can learn to break a freeze with practice.
- Fight Theory: There has been a critical lack of research invested in all areas of self-defense for women, parents, pregnant women, and the disabled. There is really no way to legally (or ethically) reproduce the most dangerous aspects of being pregnant or raped in a controlled environment. We must form our own strategies.

- The Seven Rules of Disengagement:
  - Rule 1: Escape and Evade
  - Rule 2: Set Your Mind
  - Rule 3: Gather Information
  - Rule 4: Make Panic Productive
  - Rule 5: The Best Defense Is a Good Offense
  - Rule 6: Don't Hurt Him, Stop Him
  - Rule 7: Never Give Up
- Weapons: blunt, sharp, electric, flexible, heavy, hot, slippery, stationary, projectile, improvised, weapons of opportunity. The deadlier the weapon, the more training necessary. Check your local laws.
  - Pepper spray may not work well against someone who is on drugs or highly motivated. Download the Pepper-Spray University PDF at ReimaginingWomensSelfDefense.com.
  - Firearms: get the best training you can afford so your firearm is protective and not a danger to you and your family.
- Basic Techniques and Concepts of Protective Offense: A few simple, thoroughly practiced physical techniques may be enough for self-defense.
  - Simple Multi-Purpose Primary Attack Techniques for Self-Defense, Early in Training
    - The hammer-fist uses the soft pinky side of your fist as a multi-directional pounding tool and requires no modification to load it with a weapon.
    - The headbutt is a nasty, hands-free technique that works well up close and personal when you need it most.
  - Other Techniques
    - Kicking and sweeping: there aren't many vulnerable areas on your attacker that are reachable with kicks. Only kick as a primary attack if you have complete confidence, otherwise, use it in your secondary bombardment once he is on the defensive. High kicks put you in a vulnerable position, so kick at your waist-level or below. Find a kicking style that speaks to you.

Chapter 9: The Self-Defense Continuum, Stage 4

- Elbows and knees have limited target capabilities and require power. With more training elbow strikes may be useful for getting an attacker into a stand-up joint lock.
- Biting and eye gouging don't take a lot of training, but they do require a high degree of urgency, and a strong stomach. Eye gouging is only advisable as a primary attack if you find your hands near his head already.
- Chokes: The blood choke occurs at the sides of the neck, cuts off blood to the brain and takes about five to twenty seconds to work. The air choke closes the trachea or larynx, cutting off air, and takes from ten to thirty seconds or more. The air choke is dangerous to practice due to the serious risk of crushing the trachea. Side-of-the-neck blood chokes are likely to require less strength and to be faster and more reliable in self-defense.
- Joint locks are a specialty that take years and dedication to master. The one exception might be finger locks. A few good lessons may be enough to put these into practice.
- Bonus technique: the tactical or power slap to the ear is a possible primary and excellent secondary attack. My main concern is that it will be blocked. However, if you succeed it can be so devastating as to entirely disable most people.

o On being grabbed or held, stand-up grappling, and ground fighting: Maintain distance at any cost. If you are grabbed, the options diminish and you must be brutal. Learn a few effective grappling techniques and master them.

o On footwork: In a fight you need balance and agility. Use what you already know—skills like boxing and dance give you a head start and can be adapted.

o On falling and ground-fighting: attacks on women often involve being pushed or thrown to the ground.
  - Learn multiple ways of falling.
  - Practice getting up and down as quickly as you can from many positions.
  - Always protect your head.
  - Hold your child's head in the crook of your neck to make protecting it reflexive.

- Practice on a padded surface and in slow motion, which builds muscle memory, control, and strength.
  - Basics of power generation: grounding (or rooting), coiling, and center of gravity: Learn to focus strength from your whole body into one target.
    - Grounding describes the process of softening lower joints, sinking body weight, and spreading the feet to grip the ground.
    - Coiling describes the creation of rotational force. It is the difference between hitting with a single limb and hitting with your entire body.
    - Center of gravity (COG) is as much a feeling as a place on your body. In training COG resides somewhere behind the belly button, toward center mass, or lower toward the pelvis.
    - Power generation is the synergistic process of gathering strength from the entire body using grounding, coiling, and center of gravity among other things.
  - The primary attack is a devastating surprise attack that creates an opening for you to bombard your assailant before he disables you.
- Train Intelligently—Seven Training Tips of Protective Offense
  1. Observe the Rule of Equal Motion: Practice each technique with the assumption that you have the same time-to-movement ratio as your potential attacker.
  2. Repurpose pretrained neuromuscular pathways (RPNP): Repurpose movements that are already familiar to you rather than only drilling unfamiliar movements thousands of times.
  3. Keep It Simple, Sister: Make the fighting techniques you plan to rely on simple so they are more likely to become automatic.
  4. Train Your Flinch/Flail reaction to a desired response.
  5. Prepare for Accomplices: If you are surrounded, consider learning to shoot the gap, spin through the gap, and do sufficient damage to at least one attacker. Also consider avoiding the centerline of your attacker's body whenever possible.
  6. Modify Your Training: If you only train under ideal circumstances, you will only be able to protect yourself under ideal

circumstances. Train at night, on slippery surfaces, under the influence of sleep deprivation, etc.
7. Slow Practice Makes Perfect: Doing things slowly strengthens joints and soft tissue and puts you in control. Movements you perform slowly are movements you own.

Suggested Practices

Don't forget to use the tips in Train Intelligently as concepts and guidelines for ongoing self-defense teaching and training. Here are some more specific practices to play with.

 Swing lessons: Anyone unaccustomed to hitting or specifically to being hit will have a tough time protecting themselves physically in self-defense. The first experience of impact can cause a freeze reaction and, in a real-time encounter, this could be the beginning and the end.

If you are an instructor, you can prepare new students for the shock of impact by offering simple drills that acclimate them to contact at their own pace. This may be especially important for anyone who has come to you to after a physical attack or who seems especially uncomfortable with contact in general.

Besides striking a hanging heavy bag that weighs 60 to 90 pounds in multiple ways and from multiple positions, let the bag hit back. Instruct new students to push the bag themselves and allow it to hit them. The harder or farther they push it, the harder the contact. Direct them not to stop the bag with their hands but to allow the bag to hit them from different angles. Teach them to offer up the part of their body they think will be best for absorbing impact—hips, side of the body, butt—so they learn to choose. This is a great way to introduce new students to the feeling of hitting and being hit under circumstances they control. It is also an exercise in finding balance and center of gravity in the face of an opposing force. As an added effect, the drill strengthens connective tissue by making tiny ligaments and soft tissue come out to play.

The challenge increases when someone else swings the bag. Add striking while dodging and using footwork.

Tennis anyone: This is a fun and effective way to learn footwork for a sudden, self-defense encounter. Have a training partner toss tennis balls below chest level (avoid the head). Dodging balls makes you quick on your feet, and spinning out of the way deflects impact and makes it less painful. For added fun, watch the tennis ball scene in Jackie Chan's *The Big Brawl*.

Whether you are being hit by a heavy bag or a tennis ball, always pay attention to balance. Find your center of gravity low in your abdomen. Fights are messy and there are usually things to trip over, so balance and agility are of high importance.

 Hammer-time: Practice a hammer-fist from multiple angles, not just the standard stabbing motion. Scenarios are important. Someone grabs you through your car window—imagine hammering them in the arm or neck from the driver's seat. How would you do this? What is in your cup holder that you could grab to make the strike more dangerous? Begin with your fist palm down near your opposite shoulder then strike outward on any number of angles.

You can flip the palm of your fist upward and hammer-fist from the outside of your body toward your center. You may find that it isn't as strong a strike this way but is good for twisting or tearing. What if someone is behind you? Stand with your back to a training partner or heavy bag and begin with your fist close to the same side shoulder and hammer-fist the attacker (BOB or heavy bag) behind you, aiming for the groin.

Only the groin or eyes are truly vulnerable to an empty-handed hammer-fist. You always have more protective options with something hard or sharp in your hand.

Remember to work with your flail response, then tighten up your movements and focus on accuracy and power generation. Try multiple applications until the hammer-fist becomes a technique you can depend on from almost any position.

 Become a bouncer: Practice using the momentum of a fall to carry you back onto your feet. Get down to the floor and back up from multiple positions. Learn to bounce.

In a fight, you may fall or be pushed. If you're down when you don't want to be, you will feel vulnerable and be obsessed with

Chapter 9: The Self-Defense Continuum, Stage 4

getting onto your feet again. As erect, bipedal creatures, we need to be in control of our ability to get up. Use the concepts from the section on falling, and do your own research. Invent your own creative ways of getting up and down that work for your body. If you had to fall, how would you want to do it? Would you choose to land on your knees or your butt? Always protect your head from hitting the ground and from being attacked as you rise. Practice falling in slow motion on a padded surface.

If you have a baby, put a doll in your arms or in a carrier and figure out how to fall and get back up safely. If your wheelchair is pushed over, can you get back in? Can you do it with a child in your arms if necessary? Are there other things you can practice that will build muscle and make you feel more confident? If you need someone to spot you, find a partner. Look up martial artist and conflict analyst Erik Kondo, who does more things in a wheelchair than most people do out of one.

 Choose your weapon and practice with it. Figure out what you are most comfortable carrying and using and be sure it is legal. It's not necessary to buy anything expensive, but do make sure what you plan to protect yourself with is dependable. Practice with several different items until you settle on one or two. Pound pens, pencils, and medium-to-small screwdrivers into a piece of wood and see how it feels. If you like pepper spray, buy one that comes with an inert spray and test it. See how far it goes, how long it lasts, and how quickly you can release the safety. To reiterate, the reuseable, cylindrical kubotan-style metal sprays give you a secondary weapon—a hard metal object to strike with if you run out of spray or the attacker is immune. I also like the thumb safety release of these and that the spray is easier to direct and harder to accidentally deploy than the usual forefinger kinds. Make sure you practice with whatever you decide to use to protect yourself.

 Dress to kill: Make your chosen weapon part of your wardrobe. This is much simpler to do if you wear clothing with pockets. Streamlined outfits are more difficult, and purses can be tough to find things in. You want to be able to access your protective weapon in different outfits in any season. Just carrying a protective weapon isn't enough; you must be able to access it in a pinch

201

or it will be of no use to you when you need it. Think of your protective weapons as your claws—they can be in or out, but are always accessible.

Find items that attach to your keychain, have clips, or are comfortable tucked into boots. If you are tending to a kid in a carrier or stroller, make sure your weapon is accessible to you but not to your toddler or baby! Don't leave weapons in strollers. This is where distraction and human fallibility cause trouble. You really need to work these things out or your safety program could end up being a danger to you or your family.

 Practice your quick-draw: Once you have chosen a few weapons and places to carry them, try accessing them quickly. Time yourself while walking or sitting. Can you quick-draw seated in your car, in a confined space, or bundled up in winter clothing? If one arm is trapped, can you access and deploy the weapon with your free hand? If one hand is injured, will you be able to use your non-dominant hand?

 Be law-full: Inform yourself about self-defense statutes and laws in your home state whether or not you intend to carry a weapon or keep one at home. Read chapter 1 of *Facing Violence*, by Rory Miller.

 Doggy-style: Roughhouse with a big dog. This is great way to experience movement and timing. It's also fun and good exercise for you and the dog. Use your forearms at the dog's neck to turn her body, post her head down or away from you, redirect her hindquarters, and see how you can control motion. Do all this gently since you can accidently damage the dog. Respect the dog you're playing with. Figure out how to gain control of the dangerous parts. If you raise the level of play with the wrong animal, the game can get out of hand. This exercise doesn't mimic human fighting, but it can help us understand certain dynamics of physical contact.

CHAPTER 10

The Self-Defense Continuum, Stage 5— Debrief After the Reaction

SDC Stage 5: Debrief/Reaction

As self-defense analysts, and instructors, we always need to exercise discretion and sensitivity in the face of traumatized individuals. We may also need basic tools to assist those who have suffered horrific ordeals to ease back into a sense of control and safety. This requires us to care enough to look at every piece of the puzzle.

Debrief is the final "D" of Erik Kondo's Five Ds of Self-Defense. The word "debrief" describes the act of gathering information about a completed, usually recent, undertaking or event. Reaction is the final stage of the Five Stages of Violent Crime and refers to a criminal's state of mind once he has committed the act that was the primary focus of his crime. As regards the Self-Defense Continuum, it also refers to your own state of mind.

The moment of attack changes the minutes and years that follow. Let's look at the point during an attack when debriefing becomes possible.

You have just been attacked. Your assailant is still present and has not yet decided how he feels about what he's done, He may be hearing voices in his head—his own, telling him to kill you, and his mother's, telling him to be a good boy.

Five Stages of Violent Crime creator Marc MacYoung makes the point that a rapist who finds himself insufficiently empowered by the act is likely to become violent and that up to 80 percent of serious physical injuries occur after the rape. So long as the assailant is in your presence, you are at risk. Post-attack emotions run high, and a criminal's erratic and unpredictable behavior means almost anything can happen. I've heard accounts of victims pretending to be fine and hanging out with the rapist, even cooking for them and surviving, or of attackers becoming sleepy and providing their victims an opening to escape. An attacker may not have planned to kill you and change his mind, or it may go the other way. We may have an obvious opening to escape and find ourselves unable to move. We are looking for a foothold on a sheer rock face. If we say or do the wrong thing, it could be the last thing we do. This is a major reason we freeze.

Rape survivors who freeze tend to have higher instances of PTSD.[21] It's the intensity of helplessness that gets us—the inability to act or change our circumstances. When we exhaust all resources and finally give up, the brutal reality of waiting for whatever may come or living with the feeling that we did nothing becomes ever present.

Instructors must understand this. It goes to the magnitude of a person coming to us for training and the responsibility to observe, to

---

21 Anna Tiihonen Möller, Torbjörn Bäckström, Hans Peter Söndergaard, and Lotti Helström, "Identifying Risk Factors for PTSD in Women Seeking Medical Help After Rape," *PLoS ONE 9*, no. 10 (2014): e111136, https://doi.org/10.1371/journal.pone.0111136.

exhibit calm empathy, not to judge, to help them find a new story—to help them feel perhaps that what they are learning now gives them armor, so they can heal.

Mental Models and a PTSD-Resistant Mindset

Learned helplessness is a theory that describes how a person who, following multiple attempts to avoid or escape, may perceive an adverse stimulus or situation to be inescapable even if an obvious opportunity presents itself.

Learned helplessness is often the result of a faulty mental model. Mental models are diagrams and catalogs of people, places, and things that allow us to take mental shortcuts by making it unnecessary for us to remap cognitive terrain we've already explored. In *Deep Survival*, Laurence Gonzales discusses mental models with regard to why some people, trained or not, survive emergencies while others don't. Early in the book, Gonzales talks about how mental models work: "You scour the house looking for your copy of *Moby Dick* and you remember it being a red paperback book... When you search, you don't examine every item in the house, that would be tedious..." He explains that your mental model of the red paperback allows you to screen out everything else, but that if you are wrong and it's a blue hardcover, you may not notice the book even if it's right in front of you. In other words, we get into trouble when our internal and external worlds don't match. Earlier, I used an example from *Deep Survival* where a firefighter lost in a national park doesn't make a fire for warmth because he knows it's forbidden in the park. He might have been found earlier if he had thought to break the rules. Sometimes the answers are right in front of our eyes but our mental models make them invisible.

What if we reframe learned helplessness in a particular situation as observing and waiting for the right moment? Just because we waited doesn't mean we weren't acting. How we see a thing changes our responses to it and the residue it leaves behind.

Most true emergencies cannot be recreated for training purposes. As I pointed out earlier, we can't effectively simulate a rape without it actually being rape. In martial arts, survival training, rock climbing, long-distance swimming, and indeed any extreme endeavor, we can only train for what we think will occur. When we assume we are prepared for anything, we create a static mindset and set up mental models that may block creative thinking in the future. The more set you are in your overall sense of yourself and the world, the harsher it is when those two things fail you.

Gonzales explains,

> *First you deny that you're disoriented and press on with growing urgency, attempting to make your mental map fit… In the next stage … clear thought becomes impossible and action becomes frantic, unproductive, even dangerous. In the third stage, usually following injury or exhaustion, you form a strategy for finding someplace that matches your mental map. It is a misguided strategy for there is no such place…. In the fourth stage, you deteriorate both rationally and emotionally…. In the final stage, as you run out of options and energy, you must become resigned to your plight. Like it or not, you must make a new mental map…. To survive, you must find yourself. Then it won't matter where you are.*

This staged emotional response mirrors the Kübler-Ross stages of grief: denial, anger, bargaining, depression, and acceptance.

Lots of things contribute to survival in life-threatening situations: widely varying and appropriate experience, physical fortitude, self-awareness, humility, determination, and will to live. But if you refuse to accept the situation that presently assails you, all your training and worldly experience may lead you to learned helplessness and PTSD.

The Early Debrief

Phase 1: Gather Information

While you are in the fray, you may be acting on instinct alone, riding the moment. You may be in shock, over-adrenalized, shaking, possibly vacant and detached, as if you're watching it all on TV. You must now test what you've learned in the previous chapters: break the freeze, come back to yourself, and find a way to begin strategizing.

Chapter 10: The Self-Defense Continuum, Stage 5

An early debrief can begin as soon as the incident slows or ends and you have time to take stock, check in, and try to access critical thought. You must first come back to yourself, acknowledge your predicament, and be sure you will come out intact. Begin by saying to yourself, "I am here now. This is happening. And I will be fine." Or, "I am stronger than I know and will be stronger still after I solve this problem."

Next, begin by checking in with your intuition. Can you hear it? Is it telling you anything you can use? You are not alone; your intuition is with you, actively watching out for you like a ferocious friend with very special abilities of observation and assessment.

Now that you and your intuition are on the same page, begin planning by considering conscious strategy-building questions:
- What are the immediate dangers?
- What kind of assets are available to me?
- What knowledge do I have about this person or place?
- Based on my answers to the previous questions, what are my options?

I've used this technique in multiple situations. I remember using a version of it in early childhood when my mother was sick. I was alone, and didn't yet know to call 911. I couldn't reach the lock on the door, hadn't eaten in days, and began to panic that my mother wouldn't wake up. Like a lot of traumatized children, I had an invisible friend. She would ask me questions: What should we do? How should we do it? Could we open that can of food somehow? How do we reach it? Her questions implied that I had the power to save her. This implied that I was not helpless. The human psyche is a crazy place.

Even a minimal feeling of control over circumstances may greatly increase your capacity to deal with adversity. It also gives you something to do besides panic. Anxiety and shock are dangers in and of themselves. Sometimes they turn out to be the greater danger.

What are the immediate dangers? The dangers you face at the end of a rape, robbery, or other type of attack may or may not be obvious. Asking yourself this first question clarifies specific things to be concerned with and provides focus. Are you restrained? Blindfolded? Is a window of time closing? Are you getting farther away from a populated place? Is another criminal on his way? Did you hear your assailant planning your murder? Someone else's? Are you losing blood?

There may not be a need to articulate the answers. The asking of questions alone may be enough to turn up the volume on your intuitive faculties.

What kind of assets are available to me? Once you know the immediate dangers, catalog your assets: weapons, phone, exits, the sun coming up, a car going by within shouting distance, ways to divert attention away from you or to bring others' attention to you. Is there anything else on your side? Perhaps you injured your attacker and he is slowly bleeding but too drunk to notice. Perhaps he's so distracted by something you realize he left the gun on the table and you didn't even notice until you began asking yourself questions and observing your environment (remember mental models and Gonzales's red book/blue book conundrum).

What knowledge do I have about this person or place? You may have gathered a significant amount of knowledge about your assailant(s) without being aware of it. How dangerous are they? Do they want to let you go? Are they arguing? Are they distracted? Is their determination waning? Is one of them more susceptible to your pleas? What else do you know? Are you in a house, apartment, a car? Are you moving or stationary? Are you familiar with the area? Is it day or night? Is there a storm coming? Can you use any of this?

Based on the previous three things, what are your options? Be specific! Your primary goal is to survive, but that's too vague. Do you want to escape, find help, or disable your attacker? Each situation is unique. You can't do what you haven't thought of, or find what you don't know to look for.

Use what you find out from the first questions to come up with a plan. Figure out a way to escape, scare, fool, or incapacitate him. Use your intuition. You may have gleaned all kinds of inarticulable information, and you may already know what you need to do. There is an enlightening example of this in the first pages of *The Gift of Fear,* where a woman survives what turns out to almost surely be her planned murder by letting her intuition take the wheel.

Chapter 10: The Self-Defense Continuum, Stage 5

These strategy-building questions, or variations on them, can be practiced under less dire circumstances—when the boss calls you out in front of coworkers, for instance, or when you're late for a plane and stuck in traffic. Focus on asking multiple questions until answers come. Use this strategy in daily life to move out of minor mental freezes and into a more constructive mindset. Build the skill so it is there when you need it.

When no one is around to give you advice in the moment, you must be your own voice. Try a reframing exercise; if you know someone who is trained or who you respect, channel them. What would they do or say in your situation? Sometimes thinking outside our own perspective jogs our thought processes and causes leaps of cognition. Reframe yourself as a superhero in a temporary setback near the end of the movie. Project the most optimistic, outrageous, and audience-inspiring ending.

Channel your intuitive resources, ask questions, listen to the answers that come, gather information, and strategize. Lots of people will be happy to give you 20/20-hindsight advice after the fact, but it is all irrelevant. This is now. This is your situation and yours alone.

You are the expert in any situation in which you find yourself.
—Shihan Michelle, instructor, author

Phase 2: Assess for Injury

Before you read another word, make an appointment with your family to learn CPR and first aid from a reputable provider; the time will never be wasted. This is something we all should do every five years or so. Learn multiple ways to stop an arterial bleed: compression, tourniquet, QuikClot. There are ways to make a tourniquet with found materials. Get a few hours of training and look a few things up before you need the information.

As soon as you are able in the debrief process, assess your physical state. Pat yourself thoroughly in search of blood and pain. Move slowly and make sure everything is working well enough. Feel the places you cannot see: the back of your head, under your legs, your back. Then check your hands to see if there is any blood on them. Stop any bleeding as best you can.

If anyone else was injured and you have their consent, check them for blood and injuries as well and, if they can, have them check you. If anyone is unconscious, can't move, or appears injured, do not move them unless it is urgent that you do so since you risk doing further damage, causing external or internal bleeding to worsen, and even paralyzing them. Assess anyone who appears unconscious for responsiveness by tapping and calling to them several times. After this, it gets complicated, and you will need CPR skills. If possible, you should call 911 (in the US) and begin CPR, or find someone else who can.

Remember that calls are recorded, so be clear with yourself before you speak and don't incriminate yourself. Tell the dispatcher that you were attacked and describe your injuries. If you injured your attacker, say you were attacked and injured this person while defending yourself. If the attacker's whereabouts are unknown, be sure to tell the dispatcher or you will put yourself and the paramedics in danger.

Phase 3: Preserve and Collect Evidence

As soon as you're able, take note of anything you can remember after an assault that might help the police identify the culprit. Were there any witnesses who might have seen what happened? Did anyone use the culprit's name? If you were harmed or raped, try to abstain from showering. If you want him found, if you want to stop him from hurting anyone else, give police every opportunity to collect evidence.

In the US, each party should be allowed to tell their story. If they catch the guy who hurt you, he will be allowed to dispute your version of events. He may say you were in a relationship and you went crazy. His story may be seen as valid unless you show evidence of harm as soon after the crime as possible: torn clothing, blood, and bruises. Allow the collection of DNA.

To literally add insult to injury, there is a long-standing backlog in sexual assault kit testing,[22] shortages of supplies for the kits, and

---

22 "Why the Backlog Exists," End the Backlog, accessed June 20, 2025, https://www.endthebacklog.org/what-is-the-backlog/why-the-backlog-exists/.

Chapter 10: The Self-Defense Continuum, Stage 5

shortages of sexual assault nurse examiners (SANEs) who perform this medical forensic exam (MFE).[23]

You should never have to pay out of pocket for minimum standard sexual assault kit services. The Violence Against Woman Act (VAWA) guarantees full coverage for sexual assault kits and MFE services. Despite this, people are still sometimes charged. This could be because the practitioner isn't properly recognized by the state or possibly because hospitals don't know that you shouldn't be charged.[24] If you receive a bill after an MFE, you can and should dispute it.

As I write this, laws are changing in the United States around anything to do with women's reproductive health. This could unfortunately mean even fewer SANEs and other practitioners trained in women's health in general.

Phase 4: Seek Services

There is a saying among emergency responders: "If it's wet, it's infectious." If you've made contact with any of his blood, saliva, sweat, or other bodily fluids, go to a doctor or hospital even if you feel physically fine. Liquids have a way of getting around. Hepatitis is no fun, and neither are a host of other illnesses. For various reasons, it takes time to get results. You may need to test more than once over a period of weeks or even months. Violence is the gift that keeps on giving. You can speed the process up by asking to have your assailant tested if they catch him. This tells medical professionals what to test you for.

There are urgent reasons to endure this process immediately, not the least of which is that if you wait too long you may miss out on life- or health-saving treatment. There are windows for the effective treatment of some illnesses. Bloodborne pathogens and concussions can be covert and difficult to track.

---

[23] "Congress Moves to Address Critical Shortage of Sexual Assault Nurse Examiners; RAINN Partners on Bipartisan Legislation," RAINN, accessed June 20, 2025, https://rainn.org/news/congress-moves-address-critical-shortage-sexual-assault-nurse-examiners-rainn-partners.

[24] Amrutha Ramaswamy, Brittni Frederiksen, Matthew Rae, Usha Ranji, Alina Salganicoff, and Daniel McDermott, "Out-of-Pocket Charges for Rape Kits and Services for Sexual Assault Survivors," KFF, November 2, 2022, https://www.kff.org/womens-health-policy/issue-brief/out-of-pocket-charges-for-rape-kits-and-services-for-sexual-assault-survivors/.

Treat yourself gently. The simple things will matter more than you can imagine. Drink plenty of water, eat simple, healthful foods, avoid alcohol, which is dehydrating and disrupts deep sleep. Sleep and rest as much as you can. Without these simple necessities, bodies don't recover properly. This is where the habits you've built come to your aid.

The legal and medical processes can be exhausting and retraumatizing. Call someone for moral support, whether a professional or a friend. Cultivate relationships ahead of time. Love is a verb. As Stephen Covey says, fill the emotional bank accounts of people you care about and may need in the future by making yourself available to them.

Remember the four phases of the early debrief as GAPS: Gather information, Assess for injury, Preserve and collect evidence, and Seek services.

Mid- to Long-Term Debrief

At some point after trauma, you may need to focus on long-term healing. If you were physically injured, you may be looking at hospitalization, surgeries, and physical therapy, along with any number of modalities that add up to major life changes.

No one can tell you how to go forward into a new life. I could say, don't look back, only forward, or repeat author Laurence Gonzales's advice to make a new mental map of where you are and find yourself in your new place. But that would be disingenuous (even though it's excellent advice) because it takes a feat of inner strength to follow through with it. Recovery from physical and emotional trauma is a journey you brave in your own way. Try to find a guide. Even more than one. Somewhere, someone has been through something similar and has a perspective that could be very empowering when you are lost.

When I was competing in my early twenties, I injured my shoulder and it became chronic. No one could figure out what was wrong. MRIs showed nothing. Physical therapy didn't work. My left shoulder was tight and loose at the same time. I couldn't carry groceries or do dishes without pain shooting down my arm. I was working as a personal trainer at the time, and I don't know how I managed to do my job one-handed and in pain for over a year.

Chapter 10: The Self-Defense Continuum, Stage 5

A new trainer joined the team. He turned out to be a martial artist as well. He had studied Chinese medicine among other things and began working with me several times a week, though I couldn't afford to pay him. He put me through a battery of exercises I had never seen before, and six months later I won my toughest grand championship.

When I had postpartum depression I was stuck in a panic attack for six months. It felt like my mind and body were rejecting me. I thought I was actively dying. My midwife was no help at all; in fact, she made things worse. But a receptionist in the office who had endured a similar experience took my calls every day for months. She listened, and I knew she understood though there was nothing she could do. But it gave me the strength to get through to the other side.

These were my luckier moments. There were other times I didn't find a guide—times when I didn't look or looked and didn't find. In retrospect, a patient, knowledgeable, nonjudgmental guide made intolerable circumstances tolerable.

Now, my trauma-informed therapist, Cara, saves me every week by helping me articulate and reframe my thoughts and center myself. It took me twenty years to find her. If you're looking for someone, keep looking.

Post-traumatic stress disorder (PTSD) may set in right away, much later, or not at all. You can have been injured but felt you handled things well, be emotionally fine and never experience PTSD. Or your wellness could cause confusion and guilt and lead to depression. Guilt and shame after coming through an assault physically and emotionally unscathed, especially if someone else was injured or did not survive, are not uncommon. Survivor's guilt is a well-known effect of traumatic events and is listed in the DSM as part of PTSD.

If you think of yourself as tough or tend to worry about others more than yourself, it's possible to miss the signs of PTSD altogether and be blindsided by symptoms like sleeplessness or personality changes until others point them out.

You can recognize PTSD by multiple signs and symptoms and their pervasiveness and resistance to simple solutions. Signs are objective things others can see and name; symptoms are subjective. PTSD is not random or vague, it is involuntary and constant.

Signs and symptoms of PTSD:
- flashbacks: intrusive visual memories
- emotional flashbacks: feelings of intense distress when reminded of the trauma that manifest physiologically—pounding heart, rapid breathing, nausea, muscle tension, sweating
- nightmares, insomnia, and other sleep disorders
- inability to concentrate or stay focused even on simple tasks
- depression: normal life seems mundane and disconnected, excessive sleeping, loss of interest in your favorite things, an overwhelming sense of helplessness
- a feeling something could go wrong at any moment
- loss of appetite or overeating
- irritability, outbursts, antisocial behavior
- reclusion: the need to just be alone
- hypervigilance: being constantly "on guard" to the point of exhaustion
- an exaggerated startle response—jumpiness even over minor things
- panic attacks: physical episodes where you panic in the absence of present danger. You may suddenly feel pressure in your chest, like you're having a heart attack or you can't breathe (even though medically you are sufficiently oxygenated or even hyperventilating). You may feel light-headed or like the world is caving in around you. Many people describe it as feeling as if they are dying.

Try not to sequester yourself for too long. Others may be at a loss to help. Some may be scared by what happened and unable to face you. Sharing with others can feel scary, dirty, or embarrassing. You may have good reason not to trust people or to be too exhausted to engage. Sometimes the hardest part is just finding the energy to keep looking for clarity and peace. Choose the people you speak to carefully. Ask people to listen without judging or giving advice. The retelling and recreating of your story can be therapeutic or retraumatizing. It's helpful to have a patient, empathetic, nonjudgmental coach. But talking is not the only option and healing is not a direct route but a bumpy, winding road. There's nothing easy about the process of healing after an assault or other crime, but if you make informed choices now and surround yourself with good people, you will fare better in the event of any emergency.

Creating healthy habits before things go wrong makes healing easier. It's a lot harder to form new habits under duress than it is to continue ones that are already part of your daily routine. Start now.

A Safe Space

Feeling safe in your home and your skin can be difficult after either of those things have been violated. Actively fortifying your home against criminal entry may help you cope with trauma by giving you something constructive to do. After the initial trauma, feeling you have control and taking steps toward a goal is always better than simply waiting for things to change on their own.

I am not an authority on home safety though I've done some homework. We can all probably take a few steps to shore up home security and deter devious people from choosing to invade our homes. There are many options to choose from, not everything people sell you will work. Do your own homework. Allocate funds. Do the most important things first. The goal is to make a criminal's job too difficult—you want him to label your house too much trouble, to shrug and move on.

When a criminal, or a team of criminals, cases your house you want them to find your mastiff barking and multiple high-quality locks they can't pick because you bought them from a specialty store rather than a home store. When he breaks the window you want the glass-break sensor to set off the alarm or your dog to jump through the window like a superhero. You want them to be unable to find dark or easy access points and functioning motion sensor lighting.

If you live alone, think about finding a roommate who has a history of reliability and who you feel safe with. Go to a shelter and find and train a big dog. Nothing feels quite so safe as a trained German Sheppard/Mastiff mix who loves you, except maybe two of them. A large barking dog will deter most criminals unless they can see that he's tied up or you have the Hope Diamond inside.

Deterring criminals also means not appearing overly inviting. Don't advertise your new computer or fancy countertop kitchen appliance by leaving the box outside for the world to ogle. Don't leave ladders out that reach the second story window. Don't provide power tools that someone can use to break in by abandoning them near the garage. Don't leave ground floor curtains open so people can go shopping even before they get inside. If you live in an apartment like I did for most of my life, your tasks will be different. Landlords may need to be called to fix the hallway lighting that has been out for a week. If you live in a yurt or mobile home the issues are similar but the details are different.

A lot of this is common sense. Walk around your house, yurt, or mobile home and pretend you're a thief. Figure out how to get in. Better yet, pretend there's a fire and your child is inside. This is of course a different scenario. You wouldn't be concerned with the sound of breaking glass if you were saving someone, but the exercise may create a feeling of urgency and open your mind to the ease of reaching the window you always keep unlocked in the attic, from the lower roof of the garage. Do you have a fence around your property? Fences are great for privacy but conversely privacy is great for thieves too. Where are the vulnerabilities? What would you think about if you didn't want to be seen trying to get in. Be ruthless!

> There is no such thing as a house that is impervious. A professional can breech any home with enough time and resources. And if you make it too difficult to get in, you also make it difficult to get out. If you put bars on all the windows, for instance, you make it harder to escape in the event of a fire. The best thing you can do is raise the difficulty level of gaining access. Make breaking in too time consuming and dangerous for the criminal.

When you walk around your house looking for ways in think outside the box. Check basement entries. Yes, even those little windows you think no one could possibly get through. Think outside your realm of ethics, shoulds, and shouldn'ts. Doors and windows are not the only entry points. I'll never forget coming home to find my computer and jewelry gone. Some small person, a kid perhaps, kicked the dog-door protector in and made themselves at home. Sometimes we learn the hard way. I have a close friend who locked her condo doors religiously, so the thief came in through a sheetrock wall in her closet between the units. He was using his imagination, so should you.

You will find a list of home security tips to get you started one project at a time at ReimaginingWomensSelfDefense.com.

As regards trauma, it can be difficult for a hyper-alert mind to de-escalate at home without feeling the environment is safe. Lock doors and windows, set your home alarm. Keep a phone within reach. If you live alone, consider finding a vetted and considerate roommate. More suggestions in Suggested Practices in this chapter.

Intelligent Healing

What we resist persists.
—Carl Jung

If you suffer from any of the aforementioned signs or symptoms of PTSD, try to find effective methods to retrain and heal yourself, body, mind, and spirit. Treat yourself with consideration the way you would treat a loved one in your shoes. Martial artists, especially, are not good at this. And our harsh attitudes toward ourselves are often reinforced by those around us who may not fully understand. Go about healing from trauma with an open mind and a kind hand. Give yourself space and time. Healing trauma is like working with a small, scared animal: chase it, and it runs. It cannot be rushed; it must be gently and patiently coaxed out of hiding and convinced there is still safety somewhere.

Recovery from trauma may require more than one modality. You don't always see immediate results from the thoughtful and methodical work you do, but it adds up like the stories of a skyscraper. Stacking multiple self-care modalities can increase resilience and bolster your nervous system before, during, and after trauma. Along with a targeted search for professional assistance, you will find your way.

Journal

Journaling is a powerful yet relatively simple way to begin a self-exploration and self-care routine. Some people enjoy journaling while others are resistant. It may feel like homework rather than expression, but there probably aren't a lot of people who wish they had journaled less. James Clear, author of *Atomic Habits,* suggests keeping journaling from becoming a chore by stopping while you still have more to write.

There is something about getting noise out of your head and down on paper that can make you feel lighter. In addition, incremental change often goes unnoticed and, though you may think you haven't made any strides, a journal can help you see how far you are from where you began. Being able to track incremental changes will provide fuel and encourage you to keep at it the same way getting stronger or losing weight keeps you going to the gym. Consistent journaling is a priceless tool for you and your doctor and can greatly improve the effectiveness of therapy by helping you continue to bring up and process nagging thoughts. As soon as you put pen to paper, what is most urgent makes it to the page.

Write in your phone, computer, or iPad; dictate voice notes; write in bullet points, song, or poetry. Some of the greatest books and historical treatises began as journals.

> *Nearly everyone can benefit from getting their thoughts out of their head and onto paper…*
> —James Clear, *Atomic Habits*

Adopt a Therapy Pet

Dogs and cats aren't the only options; ferrets are lots of fun and can be very affectionate, and parrots become very proprietary about family members. It's well known that animals connect us to our deeper selves, free up stuck emotion, and supply us with love and stability. Saving an animal can save you.[25]

Spend Time in Nature

For many people, just being in nature lowers cortisol and heart rate and brings peace. Walk barefoot under the sky in the sand or grass, have a picnic, hike, or camp. Being inside too much can also have a negative effect on health for many reasons, so getting outside is doubly beneficial.

Many scientific and educational institutions as well as Chinese medicine specialists and tribal elders recommend earthing, the practice of

---

[25] If you choose to adopt a therapy animal, make sure you are allowed to keep it in your home and have the resources to care for it.

being barefoot (or wearing non-rubber-soled shoes)—which is said to rebalance electricity in the body and rejuvenate us.

We synthesize the urgently important and mood-managing vitamin D from the sun. If you are low in vitamin D consider getting a little morning sunlight (and perhaps supplementing with D3K2 according to your doctor).

Remember, this is just one small part of a larger healing strategy. It will take more than one thing to heal a complex issue like PTSD. When you aren't well, getting out of bed can be difficult, but if you have nature within reach, avail yourself. Try to get into a natural environment at least once a week, more if possible. Nature brings us back to ourselves. Your therapy pet will be happy to accompany you.

Volunteer

Volunteering is one of the best forms of therapy. If you feel like giving up on yourself, give to someone else. Assisting others in need offers a sense of purpose and helps us adjust focus to our strengths rather than pain or injury. Feeling we have been of service when we feel useless and afraid can be immensely empowering.

You might volunteer at a nursing home to sit with residents or help them with simple tasks or at a dog shelter to work with abandoned pets. If you aren't ready for emotional connection, look for places where cooking, lifting, or driving are needed. There are places you can volunteer with friends or with your kids. You might decide to become a volunteer EMT or fireman. Find your own comfort level. Be of service. Somewhere someone needs something.

Laugh

Years ago, I saw a documentary about laughter clubs in India where groups of people would stand in a circle and belt out huffs of forced laughter. Years later, Pamana Tuhon Sayoc suggested we laugh before bed for better health. There are even TED Talks on the power of laughter.

Norman Cousins, a writer, researcher, and professor at the UCLA School of Medicine, wrote extensively about how emotions, specifically laughter, have the power to change our biochemistry and promote healing. In *Anatomy of an Illness,* he wrote of his journey back to health from a nearly incurable and painful disease using modalities that included daily bouts of laughter.

It can be difficult to laugh when you feel overwhelmed and shut off from the world, but you don't have to vibrate the walls. Just watching or listening to something funny in the background may be enough to make subtle changes. Don't underestimate the power of laughter for mental and emotional well-being. Laughter clears the mind and buffers the nervous system against stress. It fuels our internal pharmacy and floods the body with oxytocin, the hormone of relaxation and security.

> *…also remember to make the children laugh, especially just before bedtime.*
> —Breyten Breytenbach, South African poet and painter

Play

You probably won't be playing shortly after a traumatic incident, but later, if you find yourself stuck in complacency, play can be a way to reconnect with yourself and others without requiring a lot of strenuous thought.

Find endeavors you enjoy and make them regular parts of your schedule. Sing and dance; music has magical uplifting and mood-changing powers. Start a garden or take up goat yoga (harder to be sad with a baby goat climbing on you) or laughter yoga (look it up, it's a thing).

Finding what works for you is the hardest part. Start with something simple and work up to a regular practice. Begin with a single-song dance party on your own; graduate to inviting family or friends over for an hour of dancing one day per week, or create a mini-disco in your unused basement (I bet word of mouth will travel). Accept a friend's invite to try pickleball. Buy a countertop ping-pong set (all the racquet sports are apparently great for cognitive function as well). Play with your kids—the more you play, the more you heal.

After a traumatic incident, some people head for physical self-defense classes, and some run the other way. If you or a student of yours finds it difficult to go back to class, it might be the perfect time to consider one of the internal arts. The thoughtful movements will improve any self-defense practice and lower cortisol in a calming environment.

Regular activity bolsters every system: immune, cardio-vascular, muscular, emotional. There is extensive research on the numerous, life-altering effects of physical activity. Physicality changes physiology and psychology. Whatever you choose, make it fun. Don't exercise, play.

Eat Beautifully

If protective offense is partly about functioning at your mental, emotional, and physical peak, nutrition is as good a place to begin as any. Modify your diet intelligently and eat the highest quality foods you can afford.

In the 80s and 90s when I competed, I dutifully carbo-loaded pounds of whole-grain pasta and bagels. I later found I have an inflammatory response to wheat, sugar, and alcohol (all forms of sugar). My son inherited the same sensitivities. Years before anyone was discussing systemic inflammation as a major health issue, I complained that my joints felt angry all the time. I had chronic tendonitis and panic attacks. I was in my twenties. I look back and wonder how many fewer injuries, surgeries, and sleepless nights I might have endured.

Functional medicine physicians like Mark Hyman and Sara Szal Gottfried warn of the dangers of sugar. The research on this is everywhere, but the world is addicted. Brain scientist Dr. Daniel Amen writes that wheat gluten causes behavior problems and panic attacks in some people, especially those with ADHD, autism, and associated issues.[26] In addition, lack of nutrition is a huge issue. Our bodies and brains cannot function or heal without certain nutrients, and there is less nutrition in our food than ever before. Poor nutrition and a diet of processed, chemical-ridden foods play a major role in the American epidemic of inflammation, anxiety, brain fog, depression, rage, low energy, and a myriad of autoimmune and sleep disorders that exacerbate PTSD and keep us sick and injured. Our bodies perform alchemy every day, but there is a limit. We can't continue to take in garbage and expect gold medals.

Most physicians hardly study nutrition at all. Get your information from multiple vetted sources or from a licensed nutritionist or dietician. Find your own food gurus. Heed author and food journalist Michael

---
26 Daniel G. Amen, *Healing ADD* (Berkely: Penguin Random House, 2013), 244.

Pollan and "eat food, not too much, mostly plants." If you take care of your body now, recovery from almost anything will be easier.

Seek Inner Peace and Stillness

I mentioned meditation earlier, but it merits at least a slightly more detailed treatment. When I was younger, sitting still was virtually impossible, and I never learned to meditate the way the monks do. Instead, I did tai chi and yoga or walked or hiked in nature. Moving meditation is excellent for stress relief and I highly recommend it. Traditional eyes-closed, seated meditation can help you get to deeper places, but it takes dedication, especially for those who are skeptical or who have difficulty sitting still.

Yoga, meditation, and breathing gurus are everywhere, and so is misinformation. Many will tell you to empty your mind, but it may be about as easy to empty your mind for twenty minutes as it would be to hold your breath that long. There are some useful starter apps, but to learn deep meditation you may want a teacher, live or online, who can answer questions and explain things in a clear and helpful way. There are many different forms of meditation, and you will have to ask around or do your own research.

Find a safe, comfortable place to sit—not necessarily cross-legged but with your back supported and your head free so you don't fall asleep too easily. Close your eyes. You might begin with a few minutes of simple yogic breathing, like alternate nostril breathing or breath of fire.[27] To meditate, simply begin to note the feeling of breath as it enters and leaves your nose and expands and releases your diaphragm at your midbody. Some meditation styles include a mantra—a single word or sound to focus softly on. You can begin by using a simple nature word like "air," "water," or "earth" to anchor you as your mind flows around it. Once you have a teacher you will be given a personal mantra. When thoughts overwhelm you—which they will—don't wrestle or banish them, simply wander back to your breath or mantra.

There are many ways to finish your meditation, but a gratitude

---

[27] Contraindications for breath of fire include: cardiac issues, back injuries, respiratory infection, or pregnancy. Consult your doctor.

Chapter 10: The Self-Defense Continuum, Stage 5

practice works well. All this means is that you find someone or something you are grateful for and spend a moment in appreciation: a friend, your child, your partner, your garden, your pet, your own resilience and willingness to keep learning. Then you open your eyes, breathe, and go on with your day.

There are lots of small changes you can make to the above recipe. This is not a meditation book, but I want to keep you from being deterred by wrong-headed concepts of sitting absolutely still and struggling to keep your mind clear—things that kept me from meditating for years. If you're hyper-active—and many martial artists are—do five minutes of yoga or some form of movement right before you meditate. This makes all the difference for me. You might simply clench your entire body three times, for five seconds each time, then release, to shake off any physical tension that might make seated meditation difficult.

Pick up Dan Harris' books *Meditation for Fidgety Skeptics* and *10% Happier*, or try *Stress Less, Accomplish More* by meditation teacher Emily Fletcher. Studies suggest the best results come from twenty minutes twice a day, but as Emily and Voltaire say, "Don't let perfect be the enemy of good."

> *Once you get the hang of it, the practice [of meditation] can create just enough space in your head that when you get angry or annoyed you are less likely to take the bait and act on it. There's even science to back this up—an explosion of new research, complete with colorful MRI scans, demonstrating that meditation can essentially rewire your brain.*[28]
> —Dan Harris, author of *10 Percent Happier*, ABC News and *Good Morning America* news anchor

If you seek out yoga, tai chi, or qigong—forms of moving relaxation—be sure to find reputable instructors. There seem to be an awful lot of McTeachers around these days. To become a yoga instructor,

---

[28] Adrienne A. Taren, Peter J. Gianaros, Carol M. Greco, Emily K. Lindsay, April Fairgrieve, Kirk Warren Brown, Rhonda K. Rosen, Jennifer L. Ferris, Erica Julson, Anna L. Marsland, James K. Bursley, Jared Ramsburg, and J. David Creswell, "Mindfulness Meditation Training Alters Stress-Related Amygdala Resting State Functional Connectivity: A Randomized Controlled Trial," *Social Cognitive and Affective Neuroscience* 10, no. 12 (2015): 1758–68, https://doi.org/10.1093/scan/nsv066.

you used to have to study under a mentor for years, but now you can be certified in a fraction of that time. You may find good tai chi and qigong instructors at your local YMCA. If there's a Chinatown nearby, check the parks for individuals or small groups of people moving in slow motion, especially between sunrise and 8 am.

Meditation in the morning and after lunch and fifteen minutes of yoga before bed help me sleep more deeply and consistently, and I rely on them. Before these modalities, I sometimes lay in bed for forty minutes or more struggling to fall asleep and woke up often.

Breathwork is having a renaissance right now. Practiced with the right instructor, it can be a miraculous way to dispel negative emotion and energize the body. As one of the few involuntary processes consciously accessible to us (blinking is the other one), we can use breathing to tap directly into the nervous system to stimulate the vagus nerve and even retrain physiological and emotional responses.

There are vastly different breathing styles, focuses, and teaching methods. Find a reputable teacher, online or live, whose sensibility feels right to you. Try several until one fits. I learned from clinical psychologist Belisa Vranich. A properly trained teacher should be able to examine your breathing and diagnose any dysfunction. If you are flattening your belly on the inhale and expanding it on the exhale, for instance, you are engaging in paradoxical breathing, which needs to be corrected. If you breathe into your chest and shoulders, you are encouraging a fight-or-flight response in your nervous system in opposition to relaxation.

You will be utterly surprised at how complex breathing is and how energizing and empowering it can be. It is not yet easy to access breathing instructors who are also trained in trauma relief for an affordable price, and breathwork is not covered by insurance as of this writing. Still, exploration can be exciting and distracting if you're stressed, and you never know what treasures you might find.

Here is one simple breathing tip: before you take a deep breath, give a little exhale. Exhaling is underrated. It's difficult to fill your lungs fully without first exhaling. Whenever your yoga teacher tells you to take a deep breath, make it a point to exhale briefly first. Try pausing for a second or more at the bottom of each exhale whenever you are trying to de-escalate your nervous system. This brief pause keeps you from rushing to the next breath and allows you to slow your breathing, which invites engagement of the parasympathetic nervous system, the system responsible for soothing fight or flight.

Habits that bring clarity, relaxation, and focus can buffer you against current and future stress and are a tremendous boon to overall health. Stillness and relaxation practices require some time to settle into. Start before you really need them.

Sleep Beautifully

It will be difficult to heal after trauma if you suffer from insomnia or your sleep is chronically disrupted. Sleep issues common in PTSD compound other symptoms like depression and anxiety and affect blood sugar, mood, energy level, and cognition. If you have suffered a traumatic incident, sleep is one of the first things to tackle.

Sleep studies are a big undertaking and may not be necessary. Subtle changes add up. Habit-stacking is one of my favorite concepts and involves stacking multiple modalities synergistically. Each modality makes the others more effective. People are unlikely to lose excess fat or gain muscle by doing one thing, and medication is rarely the best option—so it is with sleep. Before you reach for drugs, stack a few sleep hacks.

When my son was little and his ADHD was out of hand we created sleep menus—personal lists of calming modalities—and chose a few each things night. They included things like: organize my space for five minutes to clear my head, plan and prepare for the next day, journal, read or look for the next three books I want to read, take a hot Epson salt bath, enjoy ten to fifteen minutes of yoga or roll out (takes practice but feels like a massage), dry brush (look it up, it can be strangely healthy and relaxing), and play soothing nature sounds. Make a list of things that calm you, try a few, and create a sacred evening ritual.

I ought to mention that this can include sex, which releases powerful stress-reducing chemicals and improves mood. Nature really is the best medicine.

Track your sleep. You might consider tracking your sleep with a fitness tracker or smartwatch which allows you to track the effects any modality has on sleep quality.

Use a tracker with caution if you are likely to become obsessed with stats. I only use mine as a guide—a week on, a week off (too much information can be overwhelming and cause stress rather than relieve it). My son and I both tried wearing two highly rated brands at the same time and the step-counting and sleep-stat discrepancy was huge. Use the device to monitor changes rather than compare yourself to "normal" guidelines which can be confusing and discouraging.

Alternatively, keep a simple sleep journal to track modalities and results. In your journal mark the times you lie down and wake up; note how you feel both before and after bed. Manual tracking will keep you from becoming dependent on external validation which can sometimes keep you from "hearing" your own sleep and stress signals.

See Suggested Practice at the end of this chapter for more ideas.

Explore Therapy

Time alone might heal all wounds, but sometimes we need a pro in our corner. In my experience with my own early childhood trauma and with traumatized individuals as a martial arts instructor and EMT, I've found therapy to be complex and tricky. What works for one doesn't work for another, and insurance complicates matters further. Where a well-trained, empathetic therapist can do wonders, a negligent, improperly trained one literally adds insult to injury. Psychotherapy comes in various forms and can be very beneficial, but only if you find the right type and the right therapist.

Talk therapy is still the most often prescribed mental health modality other than medication and is most likely to be covered by insurance. For some, retelling and reframing their story can be healing and empowering, while for others talk therapy can be triggering and even retraumatizing. Of the talk therapy models, Dr. Bessel van der Kolk, author of *The Body Keeps the Score*, recommends Internal Family Systems (IFS) for trauma recovery. Having experienced both talk therapy and IFS-centered talk therapy, I wholeheartedly agree. IFS identifies and focuses on our multiple subpersonalities (the exile who refuse to acknowledge, the manager who keeps everyone in line, the firefighter who puts out fires and handles emergencies) and encourages a conversation with and between them to heal and connect these parts and restore cooperation and balance.

Dialectic behavioral therapy (DBT) and cognitive behavioral therapy (CBT) are effective and measurable methods of regulating emotions and changing ineffective thinking and behavior, but according to van der Kolk, they may not be as effective for deep trauma.

Eye movement desensitization and reprocessing (EMDR), havening, neurofeedback, somatics, breathwork, and Internal Family Systems (IFS) all focus on deep trauma that is resistant to standard talk therapy. These therapies are ways of retraining and desensitizing the nervous system to traumatic events to bring you into cohesion with yourself. Unfortunately, these beneficial therapies can be harder to find and get covered by insurance. Many with PTSD are finding relief from pain and resistant symptoms in psychedelics. These ancient and modern medicines are making a long-overdue come back, but only a few are legal or accessible.

Word of mouth is a good place to start. Seek recommendations of psychologists, psychiatrists, and other medical professionals from people you know and trust. There are worse ways to spend a few hours than finding good physicians for the family.

The process of finding the right therapy and the right therapist is a personal one. The therapeutic relationship matters, sometimes more than the type of therapy. You are looking for an ear you can trust, a guide to help you navigate uncharted territory. The right educated professional will help you avoid walking in circles or falling off a cliff. Friends can do some of this but not on a schedule or without emotional baggage. Trauma can take a toll on a friendship, and an impartial ear can often feel safer to share with.

I don't know much about online PTSD groups except that they exist. It's another option. If you decide to use one, please find a reputable group. There are predators online as well.

If you are having more trouble than you can handle, or you are in pain and therapy isn't working fast enough, there are prescription drugs that can help. Personally, I don't like taking medication if I can avoid it. But when I have made careful choices, I have found some drugs to be of enormous relief. Think of them as a crutch for a broken leg. When you're stronger they may no longer be necessary—though you must always taper off slowly under professional guidance. Never simply stop taking a prescription drug since withdrawal can cause mania, suicidal ideation, and other issues that may feel like they're your fault but are the result of chemical disequilibrium as your body scrambles to recalibrate.

Choose the best doctors you can find and listen to them, get second opinions when you can, advocate for yourself, educate yourself about medications, don't lean on anti-depression and anti-anxiety prescriptions as a permanent solution, and keep doing the hard work. Healing post-trauma is a process without a simple road map. You may need to take a few detours before you find the right route.

Make sure you want to heal. Trauma can become part of your identity, and letting it go can be scary. Your fragile state keeps people at a distance so you don't have to engage with the world. It becomes an excuse not to heal further.

Most importantly, surround yourself with gentle people and be one yourself. Don't punish yourself for not healing fast enough. Self-bullying will cause more anger and rebellion in the parts of you that do the work of healing. Negative training methods are ubiquitous and deeply ingrained in us. The disciplinarian stands guard to keep us in our place, subservient to our basest emotions and perpetually unchanged. Be creative instead. Train your raw emotions as you would train your beloved pet or newborn baby. Meanness causes fear and hiding, not excitement and growth. Decide that you want to heal and then see yourself as a person worth healing.

> *Don't let perfect be the enemy of good.*
> —Proverb created or popularized by
> Voltaire, possibly Shakespeare

Read

Books contain life-enhancing knowledge. Here is some recommended reading to start with.

Trauma:
- *Widen the Window* by Elizabeth A. Stanley, Ph.D.
- *The Body Keeps the Score* by Bessel van der Kolk is a seminal work.
- *Man's Search for Meaning* by Victor Frankl.
- *No Bad Parts* by Internal Family Systems creator Richard C. Schwartz is an introduction to the IFS therapy model.

Chapter 10: The Self-Defense Continuum, Stage 5

Mindset:
- *The Survivor Personality* by Al Seibert.
- *Everyday Survival: Why Smart People Do Stupid Things* and others by Laurence Gonzales. (Note: Some survival books discuss triggering events involving animal attacks and suicide.)

Meditation:
- Dan Harris' books *Meditation for Fidgety Skeptics* and *10% Happier* are perfect and entertaining intros to meditation.
- *Stress Less, Accomplish More* by Emily Fletcher is great starter meditation book. Both Harris and Fletcher's books dispel confusion and provide steps to a daily practice.

Breathwork:
- *Breathe* or *Breathing for Warriors* by Dr. Belisa Vranich, a clinical psychologist and creator of The Breathing Class. Having worked closely with her, I can honestly say Dr. Belisa's work is life changing.
- *The Breathing Cure* is another important read. Author Patrick McKeown teaches the Buteyko method of breathing, which has been known to improve performance, help with sleep, stop panic attacks, and even reduce asthma symptoms. It's pretty cool stuff. Breathwork can be as helpful as talk therapy for some people.

Psychedelics:
- *How to Change Your Mind,* by Michael Pollan, is a guide to the psychedelic revolution and can be accompanied by the Netflix show of the same name.

Food and Eating:
- *Food Rules* by Michael Pollan may be the most concise, easy-to-read book on healthy eating ever written. Just keeping it on your counter will make you healthier. If you have the inclination to delve further into nutrition, read The *Omnivore's Dilemma,* one of my favorites, also by Pollan.
- *The Hormone Cure* and other books by Dr. Sara Szal Gottfried, a Harvard-educated gynecologist who has dedicated herself to helping women overcome brain fog, anxiety, depression, mood swings, PMS, PCOS, sleep disorders, and weight disorders stemming from hormone imbalances. It's about time.

- Dr. Mark Hyman is a major player in the functional medicine movement and has written multiple books on food and eating. His podcasts are a great way to keep up with current trends in health and eating. He's an engaging personality so you won't be bored.

Habits:
- *The Power of Habit* by Charles Duhigg provides the science behind habits and sparked a wave of other books and articles.
- *Atomic Habits* by James Clear, can help you create healthy new habits and break unwelcome ones so you can become the best version of yourself.

Recap

- The word Debrief describes the act of gathering information about a recently completed undertaking.
- Reaction is the final stage of the Five Stages of Violent Crime and refers to a criminal's state of mind once he has committed the primary focus of his crime. It also refers to your state of mind. So long as the attacker(s) are in your presence, you are at risk.
- MacYoung says a rapist who finds himself insufficiently empowered may become violent, and up to 80 percent of serious injuries occur after the rape.
- Mental Models and concepts like learned helplessness clarify the way our minds work and allow us to spot unhelpful thought processes so we can change them and buffer ourselves against issues of PTSD.
- The Early Debrief begins as soon as the incident slows or ends and you can take stock.
    - o Phase 1: Gather Information. Ask yourself strategy-building questions to practice moving out of freeze and into a constructive mindset: What are the immediate dangers? What kind of assets are available? What knowledge do I have about this person or place? Based on the previous three things, what are my options?
    - o Phase 2: Assess for Injury. Look and feel for blood and pain. Identify injuries and stop bleeding.
    - o Phase 3: Preserve and Collect Evidence to help catch the culprit and keep him from hurting others.

Chapter 10: The Self-Defense Continuum, Stage 5

- The Violence Against Woman Act (VAWA) guarantees full coverage for MFE services and rape kits though there has been a shortage. If you receive a bill, you should dispute it.
  o Phase 4: Seek Services. Get checked for blood-borne pathogens right away.
- Mid- to Long-Term Debrief: Post-traumatic stress disorder (PTSD) can set in right away, or much later. PTSD is involuntary and constant (see Signs and Symptoms of PTSD in this chapter). Creating healthy habits now makes healing easier (read *Atomic Habits*).
  o Creating a safe space can distract from PTSD and provide a focus. Feeling safe at home can help traumatized people find peace. See the ReimaginingWomensSelfDefense site for ideas and checklists.
  o Intelligent Healing: Stacking multiple self-care modalities can increase resilience and bolster your nervous system before, during, and after trauma. Consider journaling, laughter, therapy pets, spending time in nature, volunteering, laughing, playing, eating beautifully, seeking inner peace and stillness, sleeping beautifully, reading, and exploring therapy: DBT, CBT, EMDR, havening, neurofeedback, somatics, breathwork, Internal Family Systems (IFS), and even psychedelics for deep trauma that is resistant to standard talk therapy. Medication may be helpful when it is truly necessary, but don't use it as a crutch to avoid doing the important work. Decide that you want to heal, and then see yourself as a person worth healing.

Suggested Practices

This chapter includes many practices to bolster us ahead of time or to help us heal from trauma or PTSD. Here are some extra details.

 Tips for sleeping beautifully. Good sleep is one of the most important healing modalities for PTSD.
- **Create a sleep menu** or consider a fitness tracker or smart watch as per the Sleep Beautifully section in the chapter.
- **Install black-out curtains** or find a soft sleep mask. Look up the importance of circadian rhythms and metabolism. The wrong kind of light at the wrong time disrupts sleep and circadian

rhythm and keeps you from producing melatonin. At least an hour before bed refrain from using electronic devices and avoid artificial blue light in general. Accomplish this by cutting electronics ten minutes earlier each night. At the very least, adjust your phone's night screen settings to the warmest color or try a pair of blue-blocker glasses. Opt for orange or red nightlights and booklights around bedtime, which also won't disrupt night vision when you get up to go to the bathroom.

- **Research low-dose bioidentical melatonin.** Melatonin is a hormone, not a drug. The suggested adult dose is often three milligrams. Dr. Sara Szal Gottfried recommends much less—0.3 to 0.5 mgs four hours before bed. She says, "This tiny dose of melatonin will cause levels to spike and then decline ... so your pineal gland will start to make more..." Taking too much melatonin may suppress your own natural production instead of stimulating it. Liquid drops under the tongue are easier for dosing and may be better absorbed. Do your own research and make sure there aren't any drug interactions with your prescriptions or other supplements.

- **Adjust your sleeping space** and make it inviting. A cool room sets you up for better sleep. Open windows in season or use a fan. Find the right mattress, pillow, and sheets. Though you can't make a soft mattress harder, mattress toppers make hard mattresses and futons softer. Many companies allow you to try a mattress for a month before keeping it. Pillows are more difficult, especially if you're picky. Sprinkle your pillow with your favorite relaxing organic or wildcrafted essential oil. Weighted blankets, based on deep-pressure technology pioneered by Temple Grandin, can soothe an overactive nervous system. Finding your Goldilocks blanket can be difficult, so be sure you can exchange any blanket you purchase. White-noise or nature sounds block barking dogs and creaky floors, things that can easily wake a hyper-alert mind. Use your phone (on airplane mode) or a white-noise generator. A fan might do the trick.

- **Make your space safe.** It can be difficult for a hyper-alert mind to surrender to sleep without feeling the environment is safe. Lock doors and windows, set your home alarm, keep a phone within reach (sleep with it on airplane mode, but make sure

Chapter 10: The Self-Defense Continuum, Stage 5

you can get back online quickly). You might also keep a weapon nearby—one that you have trained with, have made inaccessible to children, and which is not easily used accidentally. Create a comfy place for your Rottweiler, Voldemort, at the foot of your bed.

 Tips for eating beautifully. The sympathetic nervous system flight or flight response in the body curtails the parasympathetic rest and digest response. Informed eating can improve health and greatly relieve symptoms of trauma and PTSD.

- **Learn about nutrients and micro-nutrients.** Learn what fiber really does, research how much protein you need for your age and activity level.
- **Eat fermented foods** like kimchi, goat milk or dairy-free yogurt, kombucha, and sauerkraut. They feed your microbiome and boost health and immunity.
- **Avoid processed foods** for too many reasons to list.
- **Lower added sugar** to less than 25 gram per day.
- Drink your **caffeine before midday** so it doesn't interrupt sleep.
- **Chew your food** thoroughly to avoid digestive problems.
- **Finish eating at least two hours before bed.** Digestion can keep you awake and overnight is when important digestive and other health functions happen. Shoot for twelve hours between dinner and breakfast.
- **Supplement intelligently** based a dietitian or nutritionists recommendations and buy from reputable sources with temperature-controlled warehouses.
- **Find substitutions.** Love Coke? Try new healthier versions of your favorite sodas instead; they're popping up (excuse the pun) like weeds. Or make fruit- or herbal-infused water and tea. Substitute the bad with better. Do it slowly so as not to shock your tastebuds.
- **Recreate your favorite meals** in healthful ways. Never go cold turkey and overtax willpower. Love mac and cheese? Try half cheese, half cooked-and-pureed butternut squash with a sprinkle of nutritional yeast (tastes cheesy). There are more recipes for healthy, delicious food than ever before.

- Like things sweet? **Try coconut sugar, stevia, or monk fruit** (no erythritol or other sugar alcohols, which may exacerbate IBS).
- Love bread and pasta? Change it up so you don't get too much of one grain. **Try lentil, chickpea, or quinoa pastas.** Try non-grain options like spaghetti squash or zucchini noodles—with a nick-name like "zoodles," it can't be that bad. Know that nothing is better than the real stuff but you can adapt. Ten thousand years ago there was no bread and no one missed it. Too many heavy carbs can tax blood sugar and digestion. Begin by mixing half zoodles with your pasta to lighten it up.
- **Keep a food diary for a week or so.** There are lots of apps for this purpose that will tell you how much protein, fat, carbohydrate, and fiber you are taking in. Log what you eat and how you feel at the end of each meal to track how food is affecting you and to spot ineffective habits.

 Tips for seeking inner peace (like assessing your breathing and beginning a breathing, yoga, or meditation practice) can be found at ReimaginingWomensSelfDefense.com.

PART 4

THEORY AND PRACTICE

CHAPTER 11

Continuing Education

Live as if you will die tomorrow.
Learn as if you will live forever.
    —Mahatma Gandhi

You're curious about protective offense and looking for ways to explore. Maybe you've covertly considered cheating on your primary martial art style; or you've been looking for something to practice as a family, or for a way to impart some skills to your kids without them rolling their eyes. Maybe you've been injured one too many times. Here are some final thoughts and suggestions for continued exploration into various aspects of protective offense.

If you're looking to try a new style, focus on the instructor, who I find to be more important than the system. If you concentrate on seeking out reputable, open-minded instructors in several systems that interest you, you have a better chance of finding the right fit. Some instructors are also authors, and reading their work is a great way to vet them before you invest time and money. A lot of cutting-edge stuff is taught by seminar rather than class. Many seminars bring instructors from sister styles and allow you to experience a variety of training methods. Some seminars involve barbecues and other family fun, which means kids and sometimes even pets are welcome. Stay clear of any seminar that offers you a rank on completion.

You won't find all the concepts of protective offense in one place. School owners are business people who must adhere to a specific learning regimen to keep regular paying students progressing and achieving measurable results. The constraints of running a business make it difficult to creatively explore fight theory or other elements of protective offense. People won't pay for long chats about fight scenarios; they want to move.

Many martial arts will supply students with strength, balance, and some understanding of power generation in a specific, predominantly physical way. With protective offense in mind, consider some of your immediate options. Judo will primarily teach you move people if they grab you, a very useful and self-defense-applicable skill; tai chi or bagua will teach you to generate incredible force while barely moving; kali will teach you to use sticks, swords, and edged weapons in ways you can scarcely believe; hard-style martial arts like taekwondo and muay thai will teach you how to kick effectively.

The downside is the old hammer-and-nail analogy. You will learn to see a potential attack from the viewpoint of your instructor and your art. If you are not attacked the way you train for, what you learn may be of little use. In addition, none of these arts were built to teach you to protect your child while pushing her in a stroller, and few are likely to help you learn to deal with the effects of a freeze response. All of them will teach you how to do very cool things if someone attacks you in a very specific way. Choose carefully. Don't buy into everything a school sells you. Don't fall in love and stay in the relationship long after it's lost its magic. Use multiple criteria before you decide.

Visit more than one school. You don't marry the first person you meet. Shop around before you commit. Check out different arts. Watch how classes are run and how people interact.

Vet the head instructor or master. These are the CEOs; they dictate the personality and ethos of the school. Ask about their background in the martial arts. Have they studied one art or several? Single-style

Chapter 11: Continuing Education

schools offer tradition and deep understanding of an art and its culture but they are not always best for self-defense.

Experience with a single style may indicate passion and dedication or indoctrination and a static mindset. It certainly indicates only one type of experience. Indoctrination lobotomizes; it shuts down the creative center of the mind and leaves behind a devotee and proselytizer. These instructors appear to be listening but then articulately regurgitate why their style is the only way to go.

There is no clear certification required to teach martial arts. Anyone can open a school. All you need is money and charisma. Check lineage. Who have they trained with? Who are their peers? What do other instructors say about them? Observe body language, especially if an instructor is a good talker. This is an opportunity to use your protective offense skills. How do the instructors stand? Is their posture open or closed? Do they look you in the eye? Do they talk down to you or seem honestly curious about your curiosity? Do they openly engage your questions?

Ask questions. Do they discuss de-escalation techniques? How do they discipline students? What are the safety practices? Ask about injuries in the recent past, specifically head injuries and dislocations. Talk to students as they come and go. Collect phone numbers or emails in case you have more questions. Is it a beneficent and encouraging environment? Many martial arts schools follow a pseudo-military structure. Decide if that approach works for you. It may help you learn teamwork and team thinking, which can be of great benefit, or it may make you feel silenced when you are there to become more assertive.

Watch a class before you take one. Most legitimate schools will offer a free trial class. Don't get roped into buying more than a few classes at a time until you commit. Watch how the classes are run, how closely instructors observe students, how they correct them, and how the students interact. And of course, make sure what is going on excites you.

Rented spaces are usually the norm for less mainstream arts, like capoeira, silat, kali, and bagua and may change locations from time to time. In formal schools you are more likely to find taekwondo, judo, jujitsu, various forms of karate, and mixed martial arts. At a formal school, you may be asked to pay by the month, while at a rented space you may have the choice to pay class by class. Schools may also have you buy your own uniform after a few classes where less formal classes may allow you to work out in sweat pants.

Don't spend money on a bunch of equipment right away. You shouldn't need much to start. If it's a traditional school, you will probably need a uniform of some sort eventually. Be sure you plan to stick around before you buy. If it's a true self-defense class, you shouldn't even need a uniform since you are unlikely to be attacked in one. If you need other equipment, try to borrow for a few lessons before investing.

Don't drink the Kool-Aid. Nearly all martial arts schools are cults in small ways. Many will ask you to be faithful only to them and require that you don't cross-train. Avoid these schools. The relief of being part of an elite club can be addictive. Enjoy, learn, make life-long friends, build strength and experience, but don't ever let your urge to be part of a group of cool people keep you from thinking for yourself.

What follows are my thoughts specifically about how the various arts fair with regard to protective offense. It is by no means a rating system or attempt to suggest which is the "best" art—something I consider ridiculous and far too subjective. The following summary is only concerned with each art as it pertains to protective offense and the goal of protecting yourself and loved ones against an attack by assailants who fight dirty and deliberately target vulnerable people.

This is by no means an exhaustive list. No one has experience with all arts or even most. Those who spend their lives teaching and loving these arts may disagree heartily with my take. I apologize in advance. There is no one correct opinion on such personal matters. All the following arts are valuable in some way. I wish I had known about many of these when I began my journey.

Chapter 11: Continuing Education

Martial Arts, Self-Defense, and Other Alternatives to Investigate in Your Search for Protective Offense

(in alphabetical order)

Acrobatics/Circus Arts/Dance: For young children, confidence, agility, balance, strength, and flexibility are often the best precursors to self-defense skills. Sometimes endeavors other than martial arts can be better places for younger children to begin their journey of assertiveness and self-protection. If they switch to, or add, martial arts later, they will have no trouble catching up with their peers. They may even have an edge.

At SLAM (Streb Lab for Action Mechanics) in Brooklyn, New York on Saturdays, my son explored multiple modes of movement: he climbed ropes, learned to flip on giant trampolines, and played on the trapeze. Some parks and zoos have tree-top obstacle courses that are great for gaining confidence and have the added benefit of being outdoors.

For protective offense, acrobatics and circus arts may be superior to gymnastics, which can be overly regimented, competitive, and damaging to young bodies. The same applies to break dancing, or ethnic dance—emphasizing circular flowing motions and self-expression—as opposed to the magnificent but unforgiving movements of ballet.

The only con would be that any type of radical movement carries the possibility of injury. The risk might be slightly higher in competitive styles of gymnastics, but it depends on the class and the instructor.

Aikido is a Japanese martial art that differentiates itself by lack of aggression and a focus on defense and submission without the need to injure. Aikido emphasizes falling, throws, rolls, and joint locks. You may also find more traditional weapons training with a short staff, sword, or knife. One major plus is aikido's focus on multiple attackers. Another is its focus on the defense/attack as discussed in the Seven Rules of Disengagement.

Aikido can be great for children and will teach them some applicable self-defense skills like falling, rolling, and using the attacker's body weight against them, without the aggression found in many martial arts.

Cons: Though a beautiful and enjoyable practice, there is a lot of brilliant flowing and falling that can fool you into thinking the same immediate and graceful responses to your attacks will occur in the street.

Dynamic injury risk from joint-locks, falls, and rolls, medium. Overuse injury risk: medium to high.

Boxing improves core strength, reflexes, cardiovascular heath, and footwork, among other things. If you learn other strikes down the line, boxing will enhance speed and accuracy. It can be difficult for people to answer a boxer's devastating strikes. Speed is one of the best ways to produce power, especially if you're small and don't have a lot of muscle or body weight to throw around.

Boxing should probably be reserved for those over fourteen or so and should only be taught by professional instructors with an understanding of and respect for the dangers of head trauma (repetitive, jarring motions may also cause problems with growth plates in growing kids).[29]

Cons: Punching works best when your attacker is directly in front of you, which is to say, it's limited. It is not necessarily the best method of striking for self-defense purposes since even Mike Tyson shattered his fist when he wasn't wearing wraps.

Dynamic injury risk from trauma, especially to the head, is low during training, medium in practice matches, and high in competition. The risk of injury from overuse depends on training style and duration—head trauma accumulates.

Brazilian jiu-jitsu (BJJ) is one of the best-known grappling styles. Training focuses primarily on joint locks and chokes to submission while on the ground. Gracie jujitsu is the best-known BJJ style and has a strong network, which makes it easy to find.

Ground fighting can be found in other martial arts as well and is indispensable in self-defense. If you end up on the ground—which is common with attacks on women—grappling skills will help you feel less vulnerable. BJJ works from multiple positions on the ground, including one of the worst positions to be in during an attack: face down. Most people have no answer for this position, whereas BJJ has many.

Make sure your chosen style also puts time and effort into creating

---

29 "Growth Plate Injuries," Children's Hospital Colorado, accessed June 20, 2025, https://www.childrenscolorado.org/conditions-and-advice/sports-articles/sports-injuries/growth-plate-injuries/.

distance and stand-up grappling since, in self-defense, this may be preferable to wrestling an aggressive and determined assailant twice your size, unless you're extremely well-trained.

Cons: You must obviously be very close to your attacker to choke him or put him in a joint lock, and training focuses primarily on this one range, so you must be comfortable with your face in his armpit. To choke someone to incapacity may take several seconds or may not work at all, depending on the precision of your choke and the physiology of your opponent. Chokes to the front of the neck may cause quick submission from pain in training whereas in a real encounter, pain compliance is much less dependable. In a live encounter, your assailant will be moving violently, grabbing at whatever they can, and clawing and fighting—just as you would in their position—so keep this in mind while training and don't allow yourself to fall into the trap of complacency. For these reasons, choking and submission-style holds may only be advisable self-defense techniques against a larger, stronger assailant after extensive training (see the "Chokes" section in chapter 9 for more detail).

The risk of both dynamic and overuse injury is medium to high. Research is ongoing, but cognitive damage may accumulate from repeated chokes.[30] You must be comfortable with close physical contact and prepared for injuries, like shoulder dislocations.

Capoeira is an Afro-Brazilian martial art with an extraordinary backstory. It originated among enslaved Africans in Brazil several hundred years ago who, barred from learning to fight, invented a dance that served the purpose covertly. Capoeira combines martial arts, dance, gymnastics, and even singing and drumming. You "play" capoeira rather than spar or fight, which makes it great for children.

Capoeira is for people of all ages, though it is very physically intensive. It's known for its complex acrobatic maneuvers, many of which you will recognize from fight scenes in your favorite movies. Though complex maneuvers aren't recommended in self-defense, capoeira integrates them so well into what feels like a natural physical language that the flowing movements make it into muscle memory faster than most.

---

30 Lucas J. H. Lim, Roger C. M. Ho, and Cyrus S. H. Ho, "Dangers of Mixed Martial Arts in the Development of Chronic Traumatic Encephalopathy," International Journal of Environmental Research and Public Health 16, no. 2 (2019): 254, https://doi.org/10.3390/ijerph16020254.

There is often little to no actual contact in classes which, though great for safety, doesn't teach what fighting is really like. What capoeira does teach is how to fight in midrange from almost any position, something many martial arts miss.

Cons: Training is mostly limited to midrange. Complex movements for self-defense purposes may not all be useful, and the art often doesn't teach contact. Classes can be difficult to find.

Dynamic and overuse injury risk is low to medium, barring competition and depending on the instructor.

Jeet kune do (JKD) was created by Bruce Lee and is now headed by Lee's direct heir, Dan Inosanto. Lee borrowed concepts from multiple Chinese arts like jun fan gongfu (or kung fu), wing chun, boxing, fencing, judo, jujitsu, tai chi, and others. Through his work with Inosanto, Lee added aspects of Filipino arnis which includes stick fighting. JKD is one of the more well-rounded arts, is loads of fun, great for kids, and can be relatively easy to find.

Cons: Some schools emphasize repetitive drills that I find can squash creativity and adaptability. If you see classes consist more of drills than anything else, ask questions.

Injury risk depends on the instructor but tends to be lower than other arts.

Judo is a Japanese art based on the much older jujitsu. It is ubiquitous and can be found in many high schools, colleges, and universities. It may even help your child get into a good college.

Judo is a rare mix of an Olympic sport that also offers applicable self-defense skills like economy of movement, center of gravity, power generation, a variety of throws, holds, chokes, and joint locks, as well as both vertical and horizontal grappling. Judo also covers safe ways to fall. Judo is at the top of my list of styles that cover a lot of ground for both adults and kids.

Cons: As with any form of wrestling, be prepared for close physical contact and injuries like shoulder dislocations. Both dynamic and overuse injury risk may be medium to high.

Kali (Filipino), **arnis** (Filipino), and **silat** (Indonesian) are arts with many similarities that work well together and are often mixed. They take many different forms, some hard, some soft. Hard styles tend to be more linear and more focused on force and impact. Soft styles focus more on circular or spiral movement patterns and redirecting attacks, rather than stopping them.

Arts from this part of the world almost invariably incorporate the use of weapons as part of the culture: sticks, knives, swords, machetes, and improvised weapons. All of these arts tend to focus on footwork, striking, blocking, trapping, disarming, efficiency of movement, adaptability, improvisation, and mental conditioning. Many styles also focus on areas rarely seen in public offerings: situational awareness, scenario training, threat identification, and targeting for critical injury, along with other protective offense skills.

Cons: Kali, arnis, and silat are among the more useful but lesser-known arts and can be difficult to find. Classes for children may be nonexistent unless you go the private route.

Injury risk depends on style and instructor but tends to be on the lower side in training and higher in matches like stick fighting and grappling.

Kickboxing (US), **savate** (France), and **muay thai** (Thailand) are some arts that combine boxing and kicking. Many countries have their own version. Kickboxing styles are usually easy to find, fun, and great for strength and athleticism. Some incorporate elbows and knees, even throws and takedowns. Kids love it.

Cons: These are mostly hard, linear fight styles that tend to emphasize kicks to the mid-body and matches in which opponents face off against each other, which limits their applicability to women's self-defense.

Overuse risk is medium to high. Dynamic injury risk is medium in training, high in competition

Krav maga is an Israeli military art that derives from aikido, judo, boxing, wrestling, street fighting, and hard-style karate, making it a mixed art.

Krav maga is one of few arts that focus on real-life situations. It is offensive and teaches aggressive attacks to end fights quickly. It is also one of the few arts (along with kali and silat) that teaches situational awareness, threat identification, targeting for critical injury, and use of improvised weapons, among other protective offense skills. Krav maga is available for children and adults and relatively easy to find.

Cons: This art is often more linear and strength dependent. It may focus on types of attacks men are more likely to encounter than women.

Injury risk depends on style and instructor.

Kung fu and **wushu** (interchangeable terms, without going down a rabbit hole), originating in China, are arguably the oldest of all martial arts. There are many arts that fall under these headings, most of which favor nonlinear or circular movement patterns. Some arts focus on fighting, others on cultivating internal power and fluid dance-like movements. Many are extremely acrobatic and physically intensive. You will find lots of amazing weaponry, including flexible weapons like the whip chain. Shaolin kung fu is one of the first and best-known styles and originated with monks in the Henan province of China, a beautiful place I had the honor of visiting many years ago.

Cons: Without many years of practice these arts may be more dance than self-defense. Acrobatic arts are lots of fun for adults and kids, but watch out for a potentially high amount of indoctrination in some of the more ancient arts. After remaining unchanged for thousands of years, your suggestions or opinions may not be welcome.

Injury risk depends on style and instructor. Overuse injury can be high or low depending on whether your instructor has also studied Chinese medicine which is less common now with Western instructors.

Mixed martial arts (**MMA**) is best known as the style resulting from the Ultimate Fighting Championship (UFC). MMA is relatively new and incorporates full-contact sport fighting, striking, ground fighting, and grappling from BJJ. It is a brutal fighting art that is easy to find and available to children.

Cons: MMA is limited to mostly linear, power-based, arena-style fight techniques.

Dynamic and overuse injury risk is, in the short term, medium to high, and high in the long term, depending on the school. Watch especially for head injury, joint dislocations, and general wear and tear.

Simulated self-defense encounters are hands-on, "live" self-defense courses, which generally involve a guy in a heavily padded suit attacking a woman who is coached to throw a number of focused and determined techniques until he cowers on the ground. Model Mugging is probably the best known of these courses which are very empowering, enliven

Chapter 11: Continuing Education

the spirit, and teach timid or traumatized women to fight back. They also teach the barrage attack, which we discussed as a strategy after your well-chosen primary attack in chapter 9.

As a close-ended seminar, simulated self-defense courses can be extremely helpful for traumatized people and those who are reluctant to commit to a regular class. This is a great way to begin a regimen and build a comfort-level with martial arts and contact sports. I am torn between finding the empowerment aspects disingenuous yet highly necessary for some.

Cons: A man in a padded suit who can hardly move, let alone fight, is not the same as a street-wise criminal with scars on his body and desperation in his soul. While some attackers will be put off by a woman with her eyes wide, growling gutturally, ready and willing to fight, surviving an attack by a determined predator may take more. This form of training is decidedly not for children.

Injury risk, low.

> One reason some women turn to martial arts after trauma could be that practice hitting things and even withstanding being hit may help them overcome the fear of fighting back. In *The Body Keeps the Score,* Bessel van der Kolk says Model Mugging courses were shown to give longer-lasting relief to women with rape or attack-based trauma than cognitive behavioral therapy.

Systema is a Russian military art that includes but is not limited to hand-to-hand combat, grappling, knife fighting, and firearms training. I don't have any real personal experience of systema other than having trained at a class that shared a large space with a systema group for a few months. I witnessed practitioners bunched up in a tight group and slowly spinning and bouncing off one another as if at a slow-motion rave. It is one of the strangest arts I've seen, and that is apparently a common assessment. Systema may not be easy to find in your area.

There are different styles of systema and again I have a limited understanding, so I can't comment on the injury risk except to say that it apparently emphasizes psychological, physical, and spiritual health, flexibility and healing, believing that training should strengthen and relax rather than injure practitioners, which is unusual except in the internal arts.

Taekwondo (Korean) and **karate** (Japanese) are among the most popular hard-style martial arts. Hard styles tend to be linear and focus on power generation and speed. Modern taekwondo (TKD) has become more acrobatic than it was thirty years ago. TKD is particularly popular with kids. Kyokushin is a more brutal, popular, and widely available style of karate in which practitioners engage in full-contact fighting without protection and even discuss self-defense options like biting.

Cons: Many hard, linear styles are less adapted for women's self-defense and tend to be more sports oriented. Many of these styles spend more time focusing on attackers in front of them, one of the least likely ways a woman might be attacked. They also tend to be brute-force styles, pitting strength against strength. From my personal experience and that of many friends, I can say that repetitive kicking and punching against hard objects in pursuit of superior strength is a war of attrition and can have a detrimental effect on joints and soft tissue.

Dynamic and overuse injury risk in the short term, medium to high, in the long term, high.

Tai Chi Chuan (Taijiquan) is the best known of the three sisters of Chinese internal martial arts, the other two being **baguazhang**, and **xingyiquan**. These are some of the oldest arts in the world and fall under the heading of the previously mentioned kung fu/wushu. These arts teach practitioners to generate force by cultivating and focusing internal energy. The movements tend to be slow, so does progress through the ranks.

Of the three sisters bagua and xingyi are more fight oriented. Taiji is the art most likely to be found in gyms, YMCAs and park gatherings, but finding a teacher trained in the self-defense aspects can be difficult.

The internal arts cultivate health and wellness in ways other arts do not and can have an extraordinary effect on well-being, which is why they are often taught for these reasons rather than for self-defense. People report that they float rather than walk, that their pains disappear, that they feel easier in their bodies, and sleep better. I have no personal experience of xingyi, but I find that my tai chi and bagua greatly increase the effectiveness of other arts I have studied.

Cons: It takes many years of practice for the internal arts to be applicable in self-defense.

Injury risk: Internal arts are more likely to heal injuries than create them.

Team sports build strength, agility, and many other skill sets and can teach kids to watch each other's backs and put their egos aside for the betterment of the team—important concepts for children (and many adults). The coach is all important as the leader who creates the culture and sets team attitude and ethos. Make sure coaches genuinely understand and like kids, not just the sport. Some take the job just to be in charge. Any coach who berates, embarrasses, or segregates kids is a bully, not a coach. They will be detrimental to your child's ability to set boundaries and protect herself in the future.

Cons: Occasionally, bad sportsmanship, rowdy fans, and surprisingly belligerent parents.

Injury risk depends on the sport.

A Note on Kid's Classes of All Kinds

Kids aren't ready for reality-based self-defense so, depending on what art you choose classes will mostly be about strength (push-ups and sit-ups), kicking, punching, balance, respect for self and others, discipline, and the like.

The instructor is particularly important where kids are involved, and the rules for vetting adult classes apply even more strongly here. You are signing up for a sort of second family, and your child is going to spend quite a bit of time with these people. Do your due diligence since, if you realize you chose poorly, it may cause great family stress to remove a child from a class they love. Choose a well-curated class run by an instructor with experience working with children. Make sure the class is adapted to what your child wants to accomplish: fun, athletics, competition, or real-world skills. Most bullies avoid hard targets and often all it takes is posture and self-confidence.

Kids who think they can kick ass can get into a lot of trouble. If there are gangs at your child's school, what they learn at a standard martial arts class could help or make things worse. Children need to learn to stay off the gang radar. Teach them what you have learned about deterrence and de-escalation, and find an instructor who reinforces these lessons rather than contradicts them.

Some schools begin kids' classes as early as four-years-old. Mostly at that age they learn to jump, roll, balance on one foot, line up, and be quiet until it's their turn. Beware of punishments like push-ups, berating, embarrassment, and other teaching behaviors that masquerade as discipline. These usually indicate instructors without proper experience who blindly follow an ensconced and broken teaching culture. The military is an important job and some of the best people I know are veterans, but the point of military service is to create well-oiled parts that work together as one machine. That is not what most of us want for our children while their minds are developing.

Franchises run the gamut and not all instructors will be stellar. Watch a class or two or even three before bringing your child. A child who falls in love with a school is a child who can't be reasoned with. Go alone first.

Reading Nook

Family reading time is rare these days, but whether you read these books together on the couch, listen to them on a long car trip, or recommend them to your new students, these books will hold your attention and answer most of your daily life safety questions in detail.

For Parents and Families. *Protecting the Gift* by Gavin de Becker is an essential guide for parents, providing safety skills for kids; warning signs of sexual abuse for parents to watch for; kidnapping strategies; ways to screen babysitters, teachers, and schools; and a great deal more. Read it with your spouse or partner. Take notes. In addition, *The Gift of Fear,* also by de Becker, is an important book for everyone (not only women) about honoring your own knowledge, experience, and intuition and also about exactly how to do that and why. It is the only book of its kind.

Safest Family on the Block: 101 Tips, Tricks, Hacks, and Habits to Protect Your Family by my friend Jason Brick is truly one of a kind. His book is an encyclopedia of practical information about everything regarding family safety you can think of: fires, driving, school, travel, sex, and social media. And it's unusually engaging and entertaining. Buy a copy for all your friends.

For Young Men. *The Little Black Book of Violence: What Every Young Man Needs to Know about Fighting,* by Lawrence A. Kane and Kris Wilder is a rare guide to violence created specifically for young men. It covers just about everything: avoiding fights, street survival, situational awareness, de-escalation, legal implications of violence, and more. Read it yourself and give it to your teenager. I know of no other book for this age group as thorough and well written.

Bonus Reading. *The 7 Habits of Highly Effective People* by Stephen Covey is a time-tested book about mastering yourself and your interactions with others. His son rewrote the book for kids and it might be even better. I cannot recommend Sean Covey's book *The 7 Habits of Effective Teens* highly enough. It's an indispensable handbook for kids learning to navigate social interactions and should be required reading at junior high schools and high schools. You can find the audiobook read by the author and a group of teens. Read or listen with your kids in the evenings or on a road trip. My son has listened multiple times since he was nine years old, and it has molded his relationship with himself and others and demystified social interactions. Stephen Covey's version for you, Sean Covey's for your kids. Compare notes.

Playtime

One of the goals of family protection is to raise assertive, emotionally intelligent, mentally and physically capable children who are aware of their world and its inhabitants. Start them young with small challenges. Always celebrate wins, reward good behavior, downplay losses, and ignore bad behavior. As behaviorists say, "Don't water the weeds." Yelling at kids, counterintuitively, often encourages the behavior you are trying to discourage. Read that twice. Kids are hungry for any form of attention. Behaviorists tell us the aforementioned techniques encourage effective and positive behavior patterns and extinguish negative behavior patterns. Keep this in mind as you play. Here are some things you can do together.

Escape Room: Teach young kids to find all exit points anytime they are inside an unfamiliar structure (you do the same). Turn it into a game by seeing who can find the most—search for doors, windows, fire escapes, any safe egress out of movie theaters, stores, restaurants, and especially hotels and malls. Encourage everyone to look for less obvious exits (through the drywall between rooms, possibly) by suggesting that way is blocked by fire or a crowd. You will have to master this skill first in order to help guide others, though kids will surprise you with their creativity. Forget the vent; they won't support your weight (that only works in the movies).

Learn the word for exit in other languages: sortie, uscita, salida, ausfahrt! But also teach kids to see beyond those lit red signs and identify even unusual or forbidden ways out. An emergency is no time to be avoiding the sign that says, "Staff Exit Only" or "Alarm Will Sound."

Channel Your Inner Beast: Animal movement is the origin of many martial arts. Widen your younger children's movement vocabulary. Call out animal names and have them move like a monkey; do it with them and make the sounds too. Have them mix it up and create their own animals.

You'll find monkey-style martial arts in many countries like China and Indonesia. Video of these arts really illustrates how limited punching is. Indonesian silat practitioners use their legs like alligator jaws. Chinese tiger claw is full of sweeping arm movements. Encourage kids to tap into their natural instincts for movement.

Play(ful) Chess: Chess is a challenging and entertaining game that teaches pattern-recognition, critical thinking, strategy, and forethought. Chess can be an entrée into social groups and a boon to college acceptance. Start kids early. Be encouraging and make it fun! Chess isn't generally a laughing matter, but kids who enjoy themselves are more likely to continue playing. Many schools, town libraries, and YMCAs have free chess clubs for kids and adults.

Flashlight Night: Candles and flashlights only! Play games in the near dark. Tell stories. Give kids simple tasks to perform with their flashlights. Have them retrieve something from their room, or guide you to the bathroom. Send them on a treasure hunt in the dark!

This modification to normal activities can be great fun and makes a sudden blackout a much less frightening experience for children. It will also help them navigate the house in the dark in an emergency with less chance of panicking.

Have a Nice Trip! Any accident that doesn't end in serious damage is a special gift. Make children bold. Celebrate the booboos. You know the look just after the fall... *Should I cry? Or am I okay?* The answer? *Good job! Yay!* I believe more sensory information is absorbed in one second of miscalculation than in a thousand hours of normal daily living. We touch something hot and know (feel) not to do it again. These moments are life's way of educating us and keeping us out of worse trouble. Wash the cut or scrape, disinfect it, bandage it, and move on. While you're at it, celebrate all mistakes. Kids are natural adventurers. Encourage them. You can't find your calling or explore the world doing the safe thing.

> *He who never made a mistake, never made a discovery.*
> —Samuel Smiles, author, government reformer

Obstacle Course/Obstacle Tag: Obstacle courses build coordination under stress. Create an age-appropriate obstacle course inside or outside using whatever you have: toys, cardboard boxes, pillows. Be sure the surface is soft (grass or sand) or they wear protective equipment. Let kids try it at their own pace. After some practice, you might time them if they have the right temperament. Teach kids to run safely to safety. To raise the stakes, chase kids and try to tag them, but do it carefully!

Obstacle Course Rewind: Have kids try the obstacle course in reverse or while moving backward to train different muscles and skills. In self-defense situations, you might have to move backward and pay attention to what is in front of and behind you. You try it too. Running backward is an underrated emergency skill.

Running away when you're scared isn't easy, especially with things in your way. You can add to the difficulty by marking only two ways off the course so kids need to think on their feet. The ways out you've marked are the only safe exits—there are monsters any other way they go. You play too. Kids love to see Mommy and Daddy fall down!

Talk to Strangers: Caution doesn't always make us safer, yet we still mislead kids by telling them not to talk to strangers. Since strangers aren't necessarily any more dangerous than people we know, this seems like odd advice.

Teach kids how to identify safe strangers. Parents might encourage young kids to become comfortable entering a store on their own to buy milk while they wait outside or to choose an adult to ask for the time or directions. In *Protecting the Gift*, Gavin de Becker suggests that if children are lost, they should never accept help from someone who offers it. His point is that the person you choose is less likely to be dangerous than the person who chooses you. He also suggests a child choose a woman rather than a man for the better odds she will not be dangerous.

There are myriad ways to create these opportunities for children. Show trust in your child so they learn to trust themselves.

Velcro: As soon as your baby or toddler is old enough, start training her to use her arms and legs to cling to you—front and back—so your hands can be free in an emergency. If you ever need to run (or, heaven forbid, protect yourself) and your toddler can hang on, your hands will be free to open doors and dial 911.

Make sure to be on a soft surface so if she falls there are no boo-boos. Try this on the beach or in the shallow end of the pool. Help her get stronger by trying to gently shake her off. Mimic running. My son couldn't get enough of this. Be careful about head-on-head contact and take intelligent precautions.

Wild Play and General Physicality: Hard, unsupervised play used to be the norm but is now discouraged. Head trauma is clearly to be avoided, but children learn trust and consequences better from contact play than from stern faces and finger pointing. People with no experience of contact play are at a grave disadvantage in a self-defense encounter.

Social Psychologist Jonathan Haidt, who wrote *The Anxious Generation: How the Great Rewiring of Childhood Is Causing an Epidemic of Mental Illness*, talks about how we must give children more time for less supervised play outdoors in the name of brain function and proper social growth. When we protect kids from wild play, we are in many ways putting them in more danger. Wild play may also be the only thing more interesting than TV and video games in which violence is often more extreme and less instructive.

Chapter 11: Continuing Education

Social animals build bonds by playing together, testing their strengths and limits, and in doing so, they learn trust.
—From the TV show *Nature*

I once took part in an ice hockey game...that involved four thousand kids all slashing away violently with sticks and went on for at least three-quarters of an hour before anyone realized that we didn't have a puck. Life in kid-world, wherever you went, was unsupervised, unregulated, and robustly, at times, insanely physical. And yet it was a remarkably peaceful place. Kids' fights never went too far. Which is extraordinary when you consider how ill-controlled children's tempers are.
—Bill Bryson, *The Life and Times of the Thunderbolt Kid*

Meditation/Yoga: Starting kids on a meditation or yoga practice early on can give them something to go to when they are stressed. Emily Fletcher created Ziva Kids, a meditation program for children that may be the only one of its kind. Check the Ziva Meditation site and tell Z bunny I said hi.

Find a Mommy and Me-type yoga class or practice yoga at home and let your toddler copy you—or even climb on you. My son loved this. When he was four he would climb on my back while I did downward dog, then tumble slowly over my head and fall off, giggling. Yoga became a game, then a before bed thing, then something to do for strength and focus and to find peace after a stressful day. As a teenager my son still does yoga before bed. Sometimes he falls asleep on the floor and then moves to the bed without missing a beat.

The Zombie Game: In Jason Brick's book *Safest Family on the Block*, he suggests a game where adults and children identify people on the street or in the subway as those who might be trouble (zombies), provide resources, or be collaborators. There are no defined parameters, just suggestions. This is a simple thought game to help kids exercise situational and tactical awareness.

Parent Playtime

Stroller Derby: Learn to maneuver your stroller. Try variations of movement over different terrain. If you use a jogging stroller and run with your child regularly, you are ahead of the game. Whatever stroller you have, be familiar with the way it moves and its various folding and break mechanisms—know your stroller well, wheels and all. Always maintain awareness of your environment.

Try the stroller maneuvers suggested below without your child until you are extremely comfortable. Weight your stroller appropriately with a bag of rice or sand until then.

- Work up to ten-to-thirty-second sprints while maintaining control. Jogging strollers are built for this, but work with what you have. The front wheel of a three-wheeled stroller may need to be locked when moving forward quickly and this can cause an issue if you need to run suddenly.
- Practice hairpin turns around a cone or box or your bag.
- Try pushing the stroller over mud, gravel, perhaps on a hiking path, up- and even downhill.
- See if you can maintain control while pulling your stroller behind you (not downhill). Is this faster or slower and less safe?
- Explore all your options. There are no rules beyond common sense safety.
- Finally, practice getting your child in and out quickly. You may find grabbing your child and running is faster than using the stroller. This depends on your physical ability, your child's weight, and the type of stroller you have.

Carrier Concourse: Running or dodging while carrying a child in a carrier is difficult and dangerous. You can improvise a workout with a weighted carrier to get the general idea. Some carriers are very hard on the neck and back. I did everything with a soft tribal-style wrap (sold under various brand names). They wrap around your body and distribute a baby's weight evenly (it feels a bit like being pregnant, though with a particularly large baby). I loved that the wrap made the baby feel like a part of my body, which made it easier to move. Aluminum framed backpack carriers work too because they sit on your hips like a hiking pack. Carrying your child as many years as you can is a great way to gain strength since your child provides an ever-increasing load.

Securely load your chosen carrier with a ten pound bag of rice to start.

- Warm up well and try a five-to-ten second sprint. Walk in between for a few minutes and do it again. Sprinting is not jogging. Your weight should not be bouncy or jarring but directed forward so your feet push the ground away behind you. Be especially aware of the difference in balance and center of gravity or the extra weight will carry you forward onto your face.
- Practice running backward, as described earlier in chapter 9. Do it without the loaded carrier first!
- Hike with your weighted carrier or child to strengthen your whole body and increase stamina. True hiking includes rugged paths and some obstacles. Great for training, but take intelligent precautions.
- Dance with your carrier. Move freely, turn, even spin, and practice balance and sudden movement. I used to do a single-song dance party in the mornings with my son, swaying and bouncing to his favorite songs.

Play Doctor

Proper first-aid and safety kits can be indispensable in an emergency and even in daily life. A simple store-bought kit can provide a starting point, but most are greatly lacking and overpriced. If you want the best for your family, you may want to build one from scratch. Get your kids interested so they begin gathering first-aid knowledge. Make it a family affair to buy, sort, and label items.

I recommend finding all the ingredients before investing in containers. Use boxes and bags you have lying around to temporarily contain the items for each kit. Once you have everything laid out, decide between plastic containers, gate-mouth bags, backpacks, transparent silicone bags, or makeup or pencil cases for each kit and smaller items within.

Remember to replenish supplies as you use them and replace older items as they expire. Replace often-used items like flashlight batteries (they sometimes leak). I've heard from reliable medical sources that ten-year-old aspirin works nearly as well as fresh and that many over-the-counter drugs are fine several years after expiration. Any prescription drug or first-aid item you depend on, however, should never be expired.

Consider taking a first-aid course. Prepare family members and children for medical emergencies in age-appropriate ways. The American Red Cross offers helpful resources, including classes designed to help children identify emergencies and use first-aid techniques.

Below I describe four useful kits. Technology changes, needs change, and I keep learning about cool stuff, so rather than fill this book with an ad nauseum list of items and gadgets, I will explain the reason for the kit and list the most important items. You will find detailed lists of supplies and their uses at ReimaginingWomensSelfDefense.com.

Kit 'n Kaboodle

This is an emergency kit ready at home or for bug-out in the event of a power outage, flood, or other unforeseen event. Use it to resupply your smaller kits, but remember to restock your kaboodle regularly. The benefit of this is that you are always cycling through supplies and keeping them fresh.

Following are some items you might include:
1. alcohol wipes or simple alcohol hand sanitizer for wounds and to disinfect supplies
2. bandages of various sizes
3. at least one flashlight and also one headlamp (and extra batteries)
4. medications: over-the-counter like aspirin, other NSAIDs, hydrocortisone cream, and anti-diarrhea medication as well as prescription medications like heart meds and epi-pens. QuikClot is a deck-of-card-sized major arterial bleed-stopper. I never go anywhere without it. Watch a YouTube video on how to use it. It's never a bad idea to have some broad-spectrum antibiotics around in case you are hiking the Appalachian Trail, a cut gets seriously infected, and you can't get back to civilization for a few days.
5. menstrual pads and tampons for wounds as well as their obvious use
6. multi-tool with pliers, metal saw, and knife. Must be good quality. Poorly constructed versions tend to rust or break. Victorinox and Leatherman are well-known brands.

Chapter 11: Continuing Education

7. safety pins (attach a few to the zipper of your case)
8. sewing kit with a few needles, some thread, and ten yards of fishing line for fixing clothing, fishing for food, and suturing in an emergency
9. tweezers for splinters and ticks (research how to use them properly; the way you remove a tick matters! You must gently pull from as close to the skin as possible without squeezing the tick too hard and causing him to regurgitate toxins.)
10. sunscreen (preferably non-chemicals formulas in which the active ingredient is zinc oxide or titanium dioxide)
11. emergency and medical info for all family members including any allergies, blood type, and doctor's contact info
12. redundant fire options: A candle or two, water-proof matches, a torch-lighter (works in wind but requires fuel), or a flint and steel (works even when wet), to make a fire for warmth, cooking, protection, and light
13. compact camp pot for cooking and boiling water
14. Compass. Should be good quality and water resistant. (Keep this in your car-ten below or in both places)
15. disposable latex-free gloves
16. first-aid manual and paper maps. Don't depend on digital versions of these things.
17. folding shovel (Keep this in your car-ten below or in both places)
18. garbage bags, heavy duty lawn and leaf, and a rain poncho. Though garbage bags do double duty, ponchos are more comfortable and cover the head better.
19. instant ice packs
20. twenty-percent picaridin insect repellant (works as well as deet which is a neurotoxin)
21. fabric or safety scissors (you might need to cut clothing to expose a wound or cut fabric into strips to make a sling or splint).
22. sharpie for marking trails in rain or leaving durable notes if you're lost.
23. signal whistle. If you're lost and tired, yelling is for help will only exhaust you further. (Keep this in your car-ten below or in both places)
24. digital thermometer

25. thin-packed reflective blankets, rain ponchos, or bivy sacs for emergency warmth (a bivy is a super-thin packed sleeping bag made of material similar to the reflective blanket)
26. solar/hand-crank radio/charger/lamp
27. water and redundant purification options (including filter bottles, filter straws, water purification tablets, etc. Do your own research)

You might include some emergency food or you might keep this separate: dried edamame (provides all macro-nutrients including protein in a long-life, one-ingredient food), nuts, and dried fruit, salt (especially if you're sweating, allays dizziness and muscle cramps in heat), or MREs (meals ready to eat).

There are several ways to contain this larger kit. A plastic container that closes securely with smaller plastic bags or boxes to separate items may be the easiest way to organize and find everything.

Since it's possible you will need to travel with your kaboodle, however, gate-mouth bags are portable and open wide like old-style hinged doctor's bags, allowing for easy viewing of everything within. Backpacks are easiest to carry but harder to find things in. If you live in an area prone to natural disasters and have had experience rushing from your home, you might want to consider a backpack with a hip strap and some kind of modular system so you can move items to different packs for weight distribution and easy long-distance portability.

Military-style packs accomplish this with webbing and molle systems but may also advertise your preparedness and make you a target of theft. If you go this route, choose plain colors over camouflage to look less tactical. Perhaps even add silly patches to make it look unassuming, even goofy. Don't buy expensive packs right away since you will likely change things around as you get to know your kits better.

Consider redundancy of necessities. Have more than one way to collect and purify water, make light, and create warmth. Keep your Kaboodle out of the way yet accessible in an instant.

The Kit-Ten (Ten-Kit)

This is your mini emergency kit comprised of roughly ten items meant to fit into a make-up or pencil case for daily carry in your purse or briefcase. I can't tell you how many times I've used my kit-ten for splinters and cuts that could have ruined a hike or a trip to the zoo. Make two or three while you're at it and give a friend (especially parents of young kids) a kit-ten for any occasion. You won't have to worry about anyone duplicating your gift.

The first ten-to-twelve alphabetized items of the kit 'n kaboodle give you a general idea of what your kit-ten might contain. You will need compact versions of some things—a mini-multi-tool rather than a full-sized one, for starters. A head lamp does double duty as a flashlight so you don't need both. Find a compact sunscreen stick. I take mine everywhere, and someone always needs it. Obviously, the medications add up to more than ten items, but finding a small, multi-compartment container for pills means it behaves as one item in your kit.

Expect to spend anywhere from $25 to $75 on your kit-ten, depending on what you have lying around the house already and the quality of products you purchase. A quality mini-multitool and headlamp can run anywhere from $15 to $40. If you want emergency gear that will work in an emergency it needs to be waterproof and durable. Go with brands you recognize. Look for single-use packets and travel-size over-the-counter medications, or be more environmental while saving money and buy tiny pill containers with compartments to be filled from regular sized bottles as previously suggested.

If you travel on a plane, remember to remove sharp metal items like tweezers and multi-tools! Give your kit a checkup at least every three to six months. Take care of your kit-ten and it will take care of you.

The Car-Ten

You could use a carton to contain your car-ten but it might be unwieldy. A gatemouth or backpack is probably easier to keep in the trunk.

This is your kit-ten for the car. Ten-plus items to keep handy if you drive often, take long trips, or have kids. Cars break down or run out of gas, we get tired, hungry, and lost on unfamiliar roads, accidents and traffic strand us, sometimes for hours. We invite problems when we are unprepared or stressed, and small issues compound. Pack a flattened backpack with a hip-strap in the car in case you need to walk a long way. You might also simply load it with your car-ten items.

I won't include items already in your kit-ten, since you have that with you whenever you leave the house (though if you're going on a long trip, you may need more of certain things like hand sanitizer).

Following are suggestions. Adapt the car-ten to your lifestyle by packing some or all of these items.

1. duct tape for fixing things temporarily (even a broken bumper), and wrapping items to condense and carry
2. first-aid kit. A car first-aid kit cab be a small duplicate of your kaboodle's first aid supplies. Never count on the ambulance to get there on time. Be sure to include items from your kaboodle that might be needed on the road like instant cold packs, especially in summer—cars can get very hot in traffic and these can be put on strategic areas like the back of the neck, armpits, and panty-line to cool blood and stave off heat stroke.
3. flashlights, plural. Add an extra headlamp beyond the one in your kit-ten, and a large, heavy-duty metal flashlight for seeing under the car or walking on dark roads. They can be used to strike an assailant as well. High-lumen flashlights can also temporarily blind an assailant. Always include the correct extra batteries.
4. fire options. At least two redundancies; see kaboodle for details.
5. food. Suggestions under kaboodle.
6. a few heavy-duty lawn and leaf bags
7. heavy-duty rope, fifty to one hundred feet
8. multi-tool duplicate as per your kaboodle
9. seatbelt cutter or two, close at hand
10. solar/hand-crank radio/charger/lamp. Remember this from kit 'n kaboodle. You may or may not want one in both places.
11. sunscreen (enough for the family) and hats during summer to stave off heat stroke in case you break down and need to walk.
12. toilet paper. One roll, re-rolled with the inner cardboard tube removed if you need to save space.
13. small, quick-dry, microfiber towel. This can be a wonderful thing, since dryness equals warmth.
14. walkie-talkies. High-quality with long distance range. (Agree on channels and protocols in advance so you can find one-another. Do some research.)

15. walking shoes. Here's a trick my friend and author Jason Brick got from his friend Nick Hughes: next time you buy comfy shoes or boots, add the old ones to your car-ten. If you break down and need to walk these can be lifesaving. Especially if you were wearing heels when you broke down.
16. warmth. Reflective heat blankets as in your kaboodle or bivy sacks since you may only have one in your kit-ten. An old wool blanket will also do nicely. They take up more space, but they dry quickly and keep you warm even when wet—that's the magic of wool.
17. water. Small bottles or a gallon jug of water changed out, especially during summer (plastic leaches into water, especially in heat, or find boxed water instead). Also, purification options as in the kit 'n kaboodle.
18. window-breaker for escaping a car if the doors won't open

Extras to Consider:
1. car battery charger. Expensive, but a big deal if your automatic car dies (if you drive manual like I do, you probably don't need one).
2. tire inflator from a reputable company. (Make sure it's powerful enough for your tires, but not so powerful it will blow the fuse in your car as happened to me twice.)
3. warm- or cool-weather clothes for each family member. Change as appropriate for the season. Synthetics, wool, or silk for winter, not cotton.

Naturally, your vehicle already contains these required car items: fire extinguisher, jack, jumper cables, reflective safety vest (which costs about two bucks and can save your life on the highway at night), road flares (use only in the absence of hazardous materials like leaking gas!), spare tire, tire chains or snow tires (if your area experiences cold winters), windshield scraper with a snow brush on one end.

Don't forget the Fuel Rule—fill 'er up! When I was an EMT we were strictly held to two-thirds "tank" gas or electric. You don't have to hold to this high standard, but I try not to fall below half a tank. Never be stranded.

The Kid-Ten

Label a pencil case ICE ("in case of emergency") or something that makes sense to your family, add the items below and discuss them with your child. Tuck the kit in a pocket of your child's backpack, perhaps with a note from you (if they are of reading age) reminding them of the simple details of how and when to use each item.

Your child may forget to tell you they ate the emergency food or used all the bandages playing with friends, so check the kit daily or weekly and restock, same as you would with your kit-ten.

This is a modular kit you can add to as they grow. By the time they get to high school they will be ready for a kit-ten, though, without any sharp items.

> *First we need to stop the bleeding, then clean, then disinfect, then bandage.... I skateboard. Trust me.*
> —Mad Max, *Stranger Things*

Toddlers

1. adhesive bandages—find some with your child's favorite cartoon characters or superheroes on them, maybe a few plain ones as well, so they don't all get used for fun.
2. cash—a few dollars and a few quarters. You can even get your toddler a little wallet or purse so he feels like a big boy. Even a little cash can come in handy in a pinch for vending machines and water.
3. Lip balm for lips and cheeks (with or without non-chemical sunscreen).
4. a small package of gentle cleansing wipes your child can use if they feel sticky and there's no soap and water. Always encourage the soap and water first.
5. pack of tissues. Good for runny noses and use as toilet paper if your child gets stuck in a restroom without TP.
6. mini-LED flashlight. Tiny, inexpensive, and can be clipped to anything. No big deal if it gets lost. In the event of a school blackout, she'll feel the power of her preparedness, be less afraid, and might even be of help. Caveat: make it clear she must never use it

Chapter 11: Continuing Education

in a cover-in-place, lockdown situation, even if it's a drill. If you're concerned about this, exclude it.

7. food in the form of a non-favorite protein bar so it won't disappear right away. Should preferably include non-trans fats and at least some protein. Carbohydrate-heavy bars may leave her hungry again in no time.

> My son was at a baseball game with his day camp. They forgot to feed the kids beforehand and the staff didn't have money for food. My son didn't eat lunch for eight hours until he got back to school at 4 pm. He was seven years old.

8. information card (preferably laminated and with sharp edges rounded) with your child's blood type, allergies, insurance information, primary care physician, and parent's names and numbers. No addresses. Hole punch it and attach it to the kit.
9. small, foldable water bottle. A folding bottle doesn't take up space or weigh anything when empty, and your child can fill it up from a bathroom sink if need be. (These bottles can be difficult to keep clean. Fill with some white vinegar, shake and leave for fifteen minutes before shaking again and rinsing. Never store capped while wet or mold and biofilm may grow.)

> To add insult to injury, the same day my son didn't eat, the baseball stadium ran out of water. It was the first heat wave of summer. Some kids were on the verge of heat exhaustion. It nearly became dangerous, and they had to leave at half-time. Bad planning. Parents can't always be there to save the day.

As your child grows you can add to her toddler kid-ten. Here are suggestions for school-aged kids, six to nine:

10. cell phone battery charger and cord if your child has a phone (in the interest of not creating more phone zombies, find a dumb phone for kids under eleven or twelve that actually only functions as phone).
11. a house key if you have a responsible child. You can buy a cartoon character or superhero key blank and have one cut specially. It

won't look like an important key to anyone else. Attach the key firmly to the zipper of the kit on a bungee so it can be used without being detached. This will keep one single key from being dropped or misplaced. As an extra precaution, make sure there is nothing in the schoolbag with your address on it in case the schoolbag or kit is lost or stolen. You never want keys and addresses in the same place, and even very young kids can remember a phone number and address with practice and encouragement (make important info into a little song for nearly guaranteed retention).
12. sunscreen stick for face and lips (if your child's lip balm already contains a non-chemical sunscreen, you might not need this).

Kids benefit tremendously from tasks that require self-reliance and responsibility. The giving of responsibility is an act of trust your children will thank you for.

A Final Word on Continuing Your Education

Choose the games and suggestions that fit your lifestyle, location, and family dynamic, and use your imagination to synthesize your own. Enjoy the process of acquiring new skills, and invite your children to love learning while supplying them with knowledge for life, safety, and self-care while you can. The rules are less important than the experiences. Learning should never be a chore. The fun stuff sticks better.

> *It is the small things—everyday deeds of ordinary folk that keeps the darkness at bay.*
> —Gandalf, *Lord of the Rings,* by J.R.R. Tolkien

CHAPTER 12

Reimagining Women's Self-Defense

To reimagine women's self-defense is to break with tradition, embrace uncertainty, open our minds to differing viewpoints, and reach for informed empowerment. It's time women's safety concerns are considered in context and women are included in the dialogue about the best ways to keep their families safe and live dynamic, empowered lives.

Here is a final model to remind us of what makes protective offense different and to help us keep track of its essential elements.

The Ten Principles of Protective Offense

Principle 1: It's Better to Stay Out of Trouble Than Get Out of Trouble. Live intelligently. Make smart decisions about who you spend time with and how you live and play. Listen to people you trust, heed your informed intuition. Become a master of de-escalation. Use the Twelve

Traits of Protective Offense to stay off the criminal radar. If intelligent living fails, leaving is always preferable to fighting. (Chapter 4: Prey or Privilege.)

> *The wise warrior avoids the battle.*
> —Sun Tzu

> *My style? You can call it the art of fighting without fighting.*
> —Bruce Lee, *Enter the Dragon*

Principle 2: To Know Yourself Is the Beginning of All Wisdom (Aristotle). Be deeply familiar with your own mind and exercise radical self-honesty. The ability to analyze and adjust behavior is a superpower. Cultivate the ability to de-escalate yourself in the name of safety. Choose your mindset, which drives your responses, but also dictates the way the world responds to you and the tools at your disposal. (Chapter 4: Prey or Privilege.)

Principle 3: To Know Your Opponent Is to Be Invisible to Him (to be unaware of his tactics is for him to be invisible to *you*). Accept the existence of the world's odd and dangerous creatures and be familiar with their devious tactics. Differentiate between social and asocial predators and between asocial resource predators and asocial process predators. Remember behavior that will deter a social predator may attract an asocial one. (Chapter 3: Where Wolf?)

Principle 4: Understanding How Crime Evolves Demystifies It. The Self-Defense Continuum (SDC) can help you make sense of self-defense and move more quickly through the OODA process, allowing you to spot incidents sooner and affording you more time for crucial calculations. (Self-Defense Continuum Chapters 5 through 9.)

Principle 5: Ignorance of the Law Will Get You into Trouble. Research and understand your state statutes concerning self-defense, force justification, and weapons. Talk to local law enforcement. Know your legal rights and wrongs. Be familiar with Duty to Retreat and Stand Your Ground laws. Don't take anyone's word for it, use an official source. (Chapter 9: Disengage the Attack.)

Chapter 12: Reimagining Women's Self-Defense

Principle 6: Your Mind Is Your Greatest Asset and Your Sharpest Weapon. In a dangerous encounter galvanize your mind, access the trigger to go from hunted to hunter. Remember the action/reaction loop and become the driver of events: attack rather than defend. To survive catastrophic circumstances with a person bent on harming you, become the catastrophe. (Chapter 9: Disengage the Attack.)

Principle 7: Perfect Practice Makes Perfect. Don't train blindly, begin with the end in mind. Find diverse and intelligent instructors you trust. Keep asking well-formed questions. Use the Seven Training Tips as a guide to keep your self-defense training relevant. (Chapter 9: Disengage the Attack.)

Principle 8: If There Is No Option but to Fight, Fight Like You've Already Won. Know in your bones that he has no chance against you. Use the Seven Rules of Disengagement to defeat a violent attack. Don't let your mind tell you it's over, don't give up until you physically can't go on. (Chapter 9: Disengage the Attack.)

Principle 9: Don't Forget to Debrief. When fight-or-flight is over, you must rest-and-digest or there will be no energy for the next adventure. Engage in strategies to help you heal intelligently, recalibrate, gather wisdom, and come through the shock of violence smarter, more resistant, and more resilient. (Chapter 10: Debrief After the Reaction.)

Principle 10: Always Be Learning. Don't study—engage, immerse, enjoy. Don't just watch or read—learn in multiple ways, then practice and pass on what you learn. (Chapter 11: Continuing Education.)

Protective offense is a paradigm that helps us see our family's safety in a greater context. Let's ask thoughtful questions and make incremental changes that greatly improve our experience of safety and our quality of life. Let's use our senses and skills in symphony, see conflict as opportunity, revel in the chess game of life, and model a resilient, self-aware, socially aware, and situationally aware life for our children so they never become victims or predators.

Self-defense looks and feels different. What now?

In the end we retain from our studies only that which we practically apply.
>—Johann Wolfgang von Goethe, German writer and polymath

The best way to learn anything is to use it. The Suggested Practices at the end of each chapter, as well as in Chapter 11: Continuing Education, provide multiple modalities, suggested reading, tools, and games to help you explore protective offense and synthesize your own concepts, questions, and techniques. When you acquire skillsets, implement new behaviors, and form new habits, big things change: you become a sought-after instructor, a more engaged and effective parent, a more secure person.

You don't understand anything until you learn it more than one way.
>—Marvin Minsky, American cognitive and computer scientist

The goal of this book is to begin a new conversation about the practice of women's self-defense. Now it's up to you. Open a dialogue about what you think self-defense/protective offense should be. Let's reimagine women's self-defense together. But be cognizant that in your excitement to share protective offense with others you, in the words of Steven Covey, "seek first to understand, then to be understood." Any discussion of changing ensconced self-defense practices, especially those rooted in thousands of years of history, can become fraught. If you step on the beliefs of other martial artists, which they have formed over many years of dedicated training, you may miss an opportunity to share information and see from a new perspective.[31] This does not mean you

---

31 There is a scale of ethics, morals, values, and beliefs. The deeper the level, the more fraught the argument. Ethics discussions can be friendly and are usually not perceived as an attack on identity the way beliefs often are. People guard their beliefs fiercely. Telling someone one of their beliefs is wrong is like telling them they're stupid or irrelevant. Use this simple model when discussing concepts of protective offense with other martial artists, and to avoid every day misunderstandings and general interactions that could push someone already prone to outbursts of anger, towards violence. Rory Miller discovered this model in his travels, but doesn't know who came up with it. He asks that if you know, you let us know so we can give credit where credit is due.

Chapter 12: Reimagining Women's Self-Defense

shouldn't open complex or difficult discussions that rattle the status quo—just do it thoughtfully.

Open your mind, seek knowledge, rethink your biases, try new things, make mistakes, be a reader, learn from everything and everyone. Let me know what you find out. The conversation continues at ReimaginingWomensSelfDefense.com.

Life is a journey. To the well-informed traveler, danger is simply a call to adventure.

Acknowledgements

Endless gratitude to Kevin Mills, my husband, soul mate, cheering section, and rock; Zane Mills VanWicklen, my son (and my sun), who keeps me honest and blows my mind every day (and who came up with the subtitle of this book when we were all scratching our heads); Russell Carmony, my best friend, humor therapist, and writing guru of so many years who always drops everything to help; to my dear friend and sounding board Rory Miller, who answers my urgent existential questions at all hours and who connected me with YMAA; to David Ripianzi, the man with the plan, and Doran Hunter, my editor and lighthouse; to the mysterious Marc MacYoung; to Erik Kondo, one of the few who gets it; to Hanna Witt Spessot, who was at my side through many iterations of the Secrets of Women's Self-Defense; Jason Brick, who encouraged me to publish this damn book already; Jennifer Ouelette, my friend with matching scars who rushed to my aid; to JB Miller, who believed in me back in the day; Belisa Vranich, who literally taught me to breathe and who connected me to important opportunities; to Ray and Jim Sellnow, who introduced me to taekwondo when I was fifteen; S. Henry Cho TaeKwonDo, where I spent my formative teen years; Rick Mitchell, who opened my eyes to the Filipino arts; Tuhon Rafael Kayanan, who introduced me to Sayoc Kali; Pamana Tuhon Christopher C. Sayoc, the genius who revealed cognitive realms of martial arts; Pamana Silak Tess Sayoc, who kept all the pieces together; Tuhon Tom Kier, who taught me to see things I didn't know were there; to Allain "Bong" Atienza for his gentle and engaging insight into the sword; Tom Bisio for helping so many on their journey into the magical internal world of Bagua; Thad Wong, Jonathan Breshin, and Kelly McDonald for their graceful instruction; Albis Suarez, whose deep, mindful, internal workouts heal my old injuries and are like serious strength training, yoga, meditation and massage in a single session; to Maher Sahabi for years of technical assistance always with a side of whimsy; Tera Warner for giving me my first big break; Cara Harmon and Leat Kuznier, who keep me centered;

Glenda Patterson, who always answers the phone; to Grace Church School's Mrs. McClaine, who made kindergarten fun when that was impossible, and Mrs. Margaret Duchovny, who taught me to tell time in first grade and seemed to know something about ADHD and autism though there were no such things; to PS 41's Mrs. Newman, protective grandmother, who saw something worthy in me; Ms. Edwards, who let me shine in drama class at IS 70, a school that was less than hospitable; faculty members of the High School of Art & Design in New York City—still a beloved haven for artist outcasts where I learned to trust myself a little more; to my theater arts teacher, Harry Lemay, who planted the seeds of meditation and taught me that teachers can be friends too, as well as Ayoka Cox, Christine Park, and Maximillian Re-sugiura who go above and beyond, and who help make education a better place; to A&D students past and present: martial artist/graphic artist Joey Docil for his steadfast friendship and brilliant drawings; Tahis Fonseca-Miranda for her steady hand in design; Rina Hyseni for turning an idea into breathtaking cover art; to Terry Lawler and New York Women in Film & Television for providing me with a community of women who support each other in the shattering of glass ceilings; to all those who have sacrificed and who continue to do the complex and sometimes dangerous work of analyzing conflict and violence; and to all women and vulnerable people who have endured violence in its many forms. We hear you. You will never be forgotten.

Bibliography

Amen, Daniel G. *Healing ADD*. Berkeley: Penguin Random House, 2013.

Ayoob, Massad. *Gun Proof Your Children: Handgun Primer for Parents*. Concord, NH: Police Bookshelf, 1986.

———*In the Gravest Extreme: The Role of the Firearm in Personal Protection*. Concord, NH: Police Bookshelf, 1980.

Bell, Paul. "The Myths of Non-Verbal Communication: Revisiting Mehrabian and Its Misinterpretation in Corporate Training." *Australian Journal of Communication* 37, no. 3 (2010): 41–52.

Bernstein, Albert J. *Emotional Vampires: Dealing with People Who Drain You Dry*. Revised and expanded 2nd ed. New York: McGraw-Hill Education, 2012.

Berry, Dawn Bradley. *The Domestic Violence Sourcebook*. 3rd ed. Los Angeles: Lowell House, 2000.

Blair, R. J. R. "Applying a Cognitive Neuroscience Perspective to the Disorder of Psychopathy." *Biological Psychiatry* 57, no.11 (2005): 119–126.

Bond, Charles F. and Bella M. DePaulo. "Accuracy of Deception Judgments." *Personality and Social Psychology Review* 10, no. 3 (August 2006): 214–34. https://doi.org/10.1207/s15327957pspr1003_2.

Bonn, Scott. *Why We Love Serial Killers: The Curious Appeal of the World's Savage Murders*. New York: Skyhorse Publishing, 2014.

Brizendine, Louann. *The Female Brain*. New York: Morgan Road Books, 2006.

Brick, Jason. *Safest Family on the Block: 101 Tips, Tricks, Hacks, and Habits to Protect Your Family*. Wolfeboro, NH: YMAA Publication Center, 2025.

Brooks, Alison Wood. "Get Excited: Reappraising Pre-performance Anxiety as Excitement." *Journal of Experimental Psychology: General* 143, no. 3 (2013): 1144–58. https://doi.org/10.1037/a0035325.

Brown, Justin C., Michael O. Harhay, and Meera N. Harhay. 2015. "Sarcopenia and Mortality Among a Population-based Sample of Community-Dwelling Older Adults." *Journal of Cachexia Sarcopenia and Muscle* 7 (3): 290–98. https://doi.org/10.1002/jcsm.12073.

Caignon, Denise, and Gail Groves, eds. *Her Wits About Her: Self-Defense Success Stories* by Women. New York: Harper & Row, 1987.

Chaney, Robert A., Alyssa Baer, and L. Ida Tovar. 2023. "Gender-Based Heat Map Images of Campus Walking Settings: A Reflection of Lived Experience." *Violence and Gender* 11 (1): 35–42. https://doi.org/10.1089/vio.2023.0027.

Children's Hospital Colorado. "Growth Plate Injuries." n.d. https://www.childrenscolorado.org/conditions-and-advice/sports-articles/sports-injuries/growth-plate-injuries/.

Clear, James. *Atomic Habits: An Easy and Proven Way to Build Good Habits and Break Bad Ones*. New York: Avery, 2018.

Covey, Sean. *The 7 Habits of Highly Effective Teens*. New York: Simon & Schuster, 1998.

Covey, Stephen R. *The 7 Habits of Highly Effective People: Powerful Lessons in Personal Change*. 25th anniversary ed. New York: Simon & Schuster, 2013.

Dahunsi, Lanre. "Martha Stout's Thirteen Rules for Dealing with Sociopaths in Everyday Life." lanredahunsi.com. July 23, 2021. https://www.lanredahunsi.com/martha-stouts-thirteen-rules-for-dealing-with-sociopaths-in-everyday-life/.

De Becker, Gavin. *The Gift of Fear: Survival Signals That Protect Us from Violence*. Boston: Little, Brown and Company, 1997.

———*Protecting the Gift: Keeping Children and Teenagers Safe (and Parents Sane)*. New York: Dial Press, 1999.

Duhigg, Charles. *The Power of Habit: Why We Do What We Do in Life and Business*. New York: Random House, 2012.

Elgin, Suzette Haden. *More on the Gentle Art of Verbal Self-Defense*. Englewood Cliffs, NJ: Prentice Hall, 1983.

Endsley, Micah. "Toward a Theory of Situation Awareness in Dynamic Systems." *Human Factors* 37(1), 32–64. https://doi.org/10.1518/001872095779049543.

Bibliography

Fletcher, Emily. *Stress Less, Accomplish More: Meditation for Extraordinary Performance.* New York: William Morrow, 2019.

Frankl, Viktor E. *Man's Search for Meaning.* Translated by Ilse Lasch. Boston: Beacon Press, 2006.

Gervasi, Lori Hartman. *Fight Like a Girl… and Win: Defense Decisions for Women.* New York: St. Martin's Griffin, 2007.

Gick, Mary L. and Keith J. Holyoak. "Analogical Problem-Solving." *Cognitive Psychology* 12, no. 3 (July 1980): 306–55.

Gonzales, Laurence. *Deep Survival: Who Lives, Who Dies, and Why.* New York: W. W. Norton & Company, 2003.

———*Everyday Survival: Why Smart People Do Stupid Things.* New York: W. W. Norton & Company, 2008.

———*Surviving Survival: The Art and Science of Resilience.* New York: W. W. Norton & Company, 2012.

Gottfried, Sara Szal. *The Hormone Cure: Reclaim Balance, Sleep, and Vitality Naturally with the Gottfried Protocol.* New York: Scribner, 2013.

Grossman, Dave. *On Killing: The Psychological Cost of Learning to Kill in War and Society.* Revised ed. New York: Back Bay Books, 2009.

Haidt, Jonathan. *The Anxious Generation: How the Great Rewiring of Childhood Is Causing an Epidemic of Mental Illness.* New York: Penguin Press, 2024.

Hare, Robert D. "Hare Psychopathy Checklist–Revised." https://criminologyweb.com/wp-content/uploads/2019/12/Hare-Psychopathy-Checklist-Revised-PCLR.pdf.

———*Without Conscience: The Disturbing World of the Psychopaths Among Us.* New York: Guilford Press, 1999.

Harris, Dan. *10% Happier: How I Tamed the Voice in My Head, Reduced Stress Without Losing My Edge, and Found Self-Help That Actually Works—A True Story.* New York: Dey Street Books, 2014.

———*Meditation for Fidgety Skeptics: A 10% Happier How-to Book.* New York: Spiegel & Grau, 2017.

Hofmekler, Ori. *The 7 Principles of Stress: Extend Life, Stay Fit, and Ward Off Fat.* Berkeley, CA: North Atlantic Books, 2017.

Kane, Lawrence A. and Kris Wilder. *The Little Black Book of Violence: What Every Young Man Needs to Know About Fighting.* Wolfeboro, NH: YMAA Publication Center, 2009.

Keller, Abigail et al. "Does the Perception That Stress Affects Health Matter? The Association with Health and Mortality." *Health Psychology* 31, no. 5 (September 2012): 677–84. https://doi.org/10.1037/a0026743.

Kendall, Mikki. *Hood Feminism: Notes from the Women That a Movement Forgot.* New York: Viking, 2020.

Lim, Lucas J. H.; Roger C. M. Ho; and Cyrus S. H. Ho. "Dangers of Mixed Martial Arts in the Development of Chronic Traumatic Encephalopathy." *International Journal of Environmental Research and Public Health* 16, no. 2 (2019): 254. https://doi.org/10.3390/ijerph16020254.

MacYoung, Marc. *A Professional's Guide to Ending Violence Quickly: How Bouncers, Bodyguards, and Other Security Professionals Handle Ugly Situations.* Boulder, CO: Paladin Press, 1996.

Maxwell, Zerlina. "How Stand Your Ground Laws Failed Marissa Alexander." *Essence.* October 27, 2020. https://www.essence.com/news/how-stand-your-ground-laws-failed-marissa-alexander/.

McKeown, Patrick. *The Breathing Cure: Exercises to Develop New Breathing Habits for a Healthier, Happier, and Longer Life.* Dublin: Buteyko Clinic International, 2021.

Michelle, Shihan. *Beyond Self-Defense: How to Say No, Set Boundaries, and Reclaim Your Agency.* Berkeley, CA: North Atlantic Books, 2024.

Miller, Rory. *Conflict Communication: A New Paradigm in Conscious Communication.* Wolfeboro, NH: YMAA Publication Center, 2015.

——— *Facing Violence: Preparing for the Unexpected.* Wolfeboro, NH: YMAA Publication Center, 2011.

Möller, Anna Tiihonen; Torbjörn Bäckström; Hans Peter Söndergaard; and Lotti Helström. "Identifying Risk Factors for PTSD in Women Seeking Medical Help After Rape." *PLoS ONE* 9, no. 10 (2014): e111136, p. 146. https://doi.org/10.1371/journal.pone.0111136.

Morris, Desmond. *Manwatching: A Field Guide to Human Behavior.* New York: Harry N. Abrams, 1977.

Bibliography

Navarro, Joe. *What Every Body Is Saying: An Ex-FBI Agent's Guide to Speed-Reading People*. New York: William Morrow Paperbacks, 2008.

Paul Ekman Group, LLC, "Are There Universal Facial Expressions?" Paul Ekman Group. October 3, 2024. https://www.paulekman.com/resources/universal-facial-expressions/.

Pollan, Michael. *Food Rules: An Eater's Manual*. New York: Penguin Books, 2009.

———. *How to Change Your Mind: What the New Science of Psychedelics Teaches Us About Consciousness, Dying, Addiction, Depression, and Transcendence*. New York: Penguin Press, 2018.

———. *The Omnivore's Dilemma: A Natural History of Four Meals*. New York: Penguin Press, 2006.

Quesenberry, Gary. *Spotting Danger Before It Spots You: Build Situational Awareness to Stay Safe*. Wolfeboro, NH: YMAA Publication Center, 2020.

Quinn, Peyton. *Freedom from Fear: Taking Back Control of Your Life and Dissolving Depression*. Boulder, CO: Paladin Press, 1995.

Ripley, Amanda. *The Unthinkable: Who Survives When Disaster Strikes—and Why*. New York: Crown Publishers, 2008.

Samenow, Stanton E. *Inside the Criminal Mind*. Revised and updated ed. New York: Crown Publishers, 2014.

Schwartz, Richard C. *No Bad Parts: Healing Trauma and Restoring Wholeness with the Internal Family Systems Model*. Boulder, CO: Sounds True, 2021.

Siebert, Al. *The Survivor Personality: Why Some People Are Stronger, Smarter, and More Skillful at Handling Life's Difficulties…and How You Can Be, Too*. New York: Perigee, 1996.

Stanley, Elizabeth A. *Widen the Window: Training Your Brain and Body to Thrive During Stress and Recover from Trauma*. New York: Avery, 2019.

Stout, Martha. *Outsmarting the Sociopath Next Door: How to Protect Yourself Against a Ruthless Manipulator*. New York: Harmony Books, 2020.

———. *The Sociopath Next Door*. New York: Broadway Books, 2005.

van der Kolk, Bessel. *The Body Keeps the Score: Brain, Mind, and Body in the Healing of Trauma.* New York: Penguin Books, 2015.

Vranich, Belisa. *Breathing for Warriors: Master Your Breath to Unlock More Strength, Greater Endurance, Sharper Precision, Faster Recovery, and an Unshakable Inner Game.* New York: St. Martin's Essentials, 2020.

Walker, Pete. *Complex PTSD: From Surviving to Thriving: A Guide and Map for Recovering from Childhood Trauma.* Lafayette, CA: Azure Coyote Publishing, 2013.

West, Natalie, and Tina Horn, eds. *We Too: Essays on Sex Work and Survival.* New York: The Feminist Press at CUNY, 2021.

Westen, Drew. *The Political Brain: The Role of Emotion in Deciding the Fate of the Nation.* New York: PublicAffairs, 2007.

Index

7 Habits of Highly Effective People, The (Stephen Covey), 251
7 Habits of Highly Effective Teens, The (Sean Covey), 251
acceptance, 38–40
Acceptance of Risk (Trait of Protective Offense), 58
accidents, handling children's, 253
acrobatics, 241
active listening, 27, 34, 59, 114
aikido, 241–242
air chokes, 175
Amen, Daniel, 221
anger signals, 87–89
antisocial personality disorder, 45, 53
arnis, 244–245
asocial violence, 51–52, 53
Attack (fourth stage of violent crime), 70, 73–75, 89, 107, 111, 123, 133–135
auditory exclusion, 145
autonomic signals, 87
awareness, models of, 31–33
Ayoob, Massad, 143, 160
baguazhang, 189, 248-249
Bell, Joseph, 79
Best Defense Is a Good Offense (Rule of Disengagement), 150–153, 196
biting, 174–175, 197
blackmail, 94
blocking, 41, 53
blood chokes, 175
blunt weapons, 156
body language, reading, 85–89
Bonn, Scott, 44
boundary-setting, 97–103
boxing, 242
Boyd, John, 75
Brazilian jiu-jitsu, 242–243

breathwork, 224, 227
Brick, Jason, 251, 256
Brooks, Alison Wood, 22
Buddhism, cultivating awareness and, 33, 34
capoeira, 243–244
Carmony, Russell, 82
carriers, baby, 257
car-tens, 262–264
Castle laws, 142–143, 195
center of gravity (in fighting), 188, 198
Chan, Jackie, 200
Channel Your Inner Beast (children's game), 252
Charm or Harm, 113
chess (for kids), 252–253
children, self-defense techniques with, 185–186, 198, 201
chokes, 175–176, 197, 243
Circle of Concern, 19
Circle of Influence, 19
circus arts, 241
Clear, James, 96–97, 217, 230
clinging (skill for kids), 254
closing (positioning strategy), 124
cognitive behavioral therapy, 226–227
cognitive bias, 40, 81, 82
coiling, 187–188, 198
common ground, finding with criminals, 40–41
conflict, managing effectively, 19–22
conscious breathing, self-deescalation and, 27
Cooper, Jeff, 32
Cooper's Color Codes, 32, 35
cornering (positioning strategy), 124
Cousins, Norman, 219
Covey, Steven, 19, 22, 212
Cox, Debo, 31

281

Crime Triangle, 69–70, 141
criminal mindset, 37–38
da Vinci, Leonardo, 80
dance, 241
Darwin, Charles, 85
de Becker, Gavin, 40, 79, 113, 130, 139, 250–251
Debrief (of Five Ds), 70, 74, 203–216, 230–231
  Early Debrief, 206–212, 230
  Mid-to-Long-Term Debrief, 212–214, 230
Decide (of Five Ds), 70–71, 74–75, 77–78, 101, 107
de-escalation tactics, 114–115
defense-attack, 152
deflection, 41, 53
Deter (of Five Ds), 70, 74, 75, 105–107
dialectic behavioral therapy, 226
Dimitri, Richard, 116
Disengage (of Five Ds), 70, 74, 75, 133–134, 269
Disengagement, Seven Rules of, 148–156, 196
Disrupt (of Five Ds), 70, 123–124, 127
Do Voices Carry?, 129–130
Don't Hurt Him, Stop Him (Rule of Disengagement), 154–155, 196
Don't WE on Me! 112
Dracula's Cape, 192–193
DuFrense, Nicole, 117
Duhigg, Charles, 230
Dyer, Wayne, 82
Early Debrief
  Assess for Injury (part of Early Debrief), 209–210, 230
  Gather Information (Rule of Disengagement), 206, 230
  Preserve and Collect Evidence, 210–211, 231
  Seek Services, 211–212, 231

ears, slaps to, 176–177, 197
eating habits, healthy, 221, 233–234
Ekman, Paul, 85–86
elbow-and-knee techniques, 172–174, 197
electrical weapons, 156–157
emotions, decision-making and, 60
equal motion, 190, 198
escalating interviews (MacYoung), 110
Escalation-Avoidance, Peyton Quinn's Rules of, 116–120
Escape and Evade (Rule of Disengagement), 148, 196
Escape Room (children's game), 252
extortion, 94
eye contact, 84–85
eye gouging, 174–175, 197
eye movement desensitization and reprocessing, 226
facial expressions, reading, 85–87
falling, 197
falling, techniques for safe, 179–187
fawn reaction, 144–145, 147
fight response, 144–147
firearms, 159–161, 196
first-aid courses, 258
first-aid kits, 257–258
Five Ds of Self-Defense (Kondo), 70–72, 74
Five Positioning Strategies, Marc MacYoung's, 124–127
Five Stages of Violent Crime (MacYoung), 70–72, 75, 204, 230
Flashlight Night (children's game), 253
Fletcher, Emily, 103, 223, 229, 255–256
flexible weapons, 157
flight response, 144–146
flinch/fail reaction, 191–192, 198
focused observation, 79–82
footwork, in fighting, 179, 197

Index

Four As, Amy Hermann's, 81–82
Four As, Rory Miller's, 50–51
framing, stress and, 21–22
Frankl, Victor, 228
Freeze, Fight, Flight, 144–147, 195
freeze response, 137–138, 144–146, 149
fringe areas, unusual behavior in, 107–109
gaslighting, 93–94
Gather Information (Rule of Disengagement), 149, 196
Gift of Fear, The (de Becker), 113, 250
Gonzales, Laurence, 31, 155, 205–206, 212, 229
Gottfried, Sara, 229–230
grabbing, 178–179, 197
grooming, 94–95
Grossman, David, 118, 144
groundfighting, 178, 197
grounding (rooting), 187, 198
guilt-tripping, 93–94
guns. *see* firearms
Haidt, Jonathan, 255
Hajee, Karim, 30
hammer-fist, 125–126, 164–168, 189, 196, 200
Hare, Robert, 46–47, 53
Hare's Psychopathy Checklist, 46–47
Harris, Dan, 223, 229
havening, 227
headbutt, 168–170, 189, 196
Health Before Vice or Vanity (Trait of Protective Offense), 58, 62–63
heavy objects, as weapons, 157
Herman, Amy E., 31
Hofmekler, Ori, 21
holding, 178–179, 197
home security, creating, 216–217, 231
hot interviews (MacYoung), 110, 124
hot substances, as weapons, 157

human brain, 25, 34
Hyman, Mark, 221, 230
improvised weapons, 161–162
inner peace, 222–225, 234
Inner Peace (Trait of Protective Offense), 61, 64–65
Inosanto, Dan, 246
instructors, martial arts; selecting, 237–240
Intent (first stage of violent crime), 70–75, 77–79, 101, 106, 111, 134
Interview (second stage of violent crime), 70–75, 89, 93, 105–107, 109–111, 119, 124, 130, 131, 134
intuition, 48, 59–60, 79, 84, 86, 92, 96–97, 101–103, 106–108, 113, 148, 207
Jackson, Kathy, 33, 155, 160
jeet kune do, 244
joint locks, 176, 197
journaling, 217–218
judo, 244
kaboodle kits, 258–261
kali, 244–245
Kane, Lawrence, 251
karate, 247–248
keys, as weapons, 125–126, 165
kickboxing, 245
kicking, 170–172, 196
kids' classes, 249–250
kid-tens, 264–266
Kier, Tom, 162
kit-tens (ten-kits), 261
Know Your "No," 100, 111–112
Kondo, Erik, 70, 72, 99, 201
krav maga, 245–246
kubotans, 158
kung fu, 246
laughter, 219–220
learned helplessness, 205
Lee, Bruce, 106, 244

legal issues, self-defense, 141–144, 195
legality versus self-defense, 135, 194
Liar's Litany, 112–113
liquid projectiles, 157–159
Little Black Book of Violence, The (Kane and Wilder), 251
lizard brain, 23–24, 33
lying, signs of, 90–91
MacLean, Paul D., 23
MacYoung, Marc, 51, 70, 204, 230
Make Like a Tree, 128–130
Make Panic Productive (Rule of Disengagement), 149, 196
martial arts schools, selecting, 237–240
martial arts training, women's; shortcomings of, 4–7
McGonigal, Kelly, 20–21, 65
McKeown, Patrick, 229
medication, post trauma, 227
meditation, 222–224, 255
Mental Models, 205–206
Messengers of Intuition, 79
Michelle, Shihan, 112
micro-expressions, 86
Mid-to-Long-Term Debrief, 212–214, 231
Miller, Rory, 26, 50, 51–52, 103, 141, 144, 160, 192, 195
mindset. *see also* criminal mindset
    basics of, 30
    importance in protective offense, 55–57
mixed martial arts, 246
modifying training, need for, 193–194, 198
monkey brain, 24–25, 26–27, 33
Morris, Desmond, 86–88, 90
muay thai, 245
multiple attackers, 192, 198
narcissistic personality disorder, 45
nature, healing qualities of, 218–219

Navarro, Joe, 90–91
negging, 93–94
neurofeedback, 227
Never Give Up (Rule of Disengagement), 155–156, 196
Newton, Isaac, 80–81
No Duty-to-Retreat laws, 142–143, 195
nonverbal communication, 60, 63–4, 82–92
Nonverbal Communication (Trait of Protective Offense), 60, 64
nonverbal deception, 82–92
nonviolent disruption, 127–130
observation, of one's own mind, 21, 30, 35
observer effect, 17–19
obstacle courses (children's game), 253–254
OODA Loop, 75
Optimal Decision-Making (Trait of Protective Offense), 60
panic, 149–150
pausing, script change and, 27–28
pepper spray, 125, 157–159, 196
permission to fight, given to self, 140
Personal Responsibility (Trait of Protective Offense), 57
personality disorders, 42–46
Physical Fence, 80, 99–100
playing, children's, 254–255
playing, healing from trauma and, 220–221
Pollan, Michael, 221, 229
Positioning (third stage of violent crime), 70–71, 73–75, 89, 93, 107, 123–131, 134
post-traumatic stress disorder, 31–32, 137, 148, 204–206, 213–214, 217, 219, 221, 225, 227, 231, 233
posture reaction, 144–145, 151

Index

power generation, 187–189, 198
pragmatism, 38–40
preclusion, 142, 195
Preparation (Trait of Protective Offense), 59, 63
primary attack, 151–152, 163–170, 189, 196, 198
process predators, 52, 53, 139, 154, 195, 268
Progressive Fence, 99–101, 103, 108
projectile weapons, 157
prolonged interviews (MacYoung), 111
Protecting the Gift (de Becker), 130, 250, 254
protective offense
  basics of, 7–8
  Ten Principles of, 267–269
proxemics, 86
psychedelics, for deep trauma, 227
psychopathy, 44–46, 51, 53, 90
Quesenberry, Gary, 82
Quinn, Peyton, 116
rape. *see* sexual assault
rationalization, 40, 41, 45
Reaction (fifth stage of violent crime), 70–71, 73, 203–205, 230
reactionary gap, 150, 152
reading, 228–230
reframing, 21–22, 28, 29
regular interviews (MacYoung), 109–110, 124
Renshaw, Samuel, 81
repurposing pretrained neuromuscular pathways (RPNP), 190–191, 198
resource predators, 52, 53, 139, 268
rooting. *see* grounding (rooting)
Rousey, Ronda, 178
Safest Family on the Block (Brick), 251, 256
Samenow, Stanton, 49
savate, 245

Sayoc, Pamana Tuhon Christopher C., Sr., xiv, 219
Schwartz, Richard, 229
script hacking, 34. *see also* social scripts
scripts, social, 25–29
Seek Knowledge (Trait of Protective Offense), 61
Seibert, Al, 229
self-awareness. *see also* Self-Awareness and Auto-Correction (Trait of Protective Offense), as conflict management tool, 31, 33
Self-Awareness and Auto-Correction (Trait of Protective Offense), 60–61, 64
self-defense, martial-arts based, 7–8
Self-Defense Continuum, overview of, 69–76. *See also particular stages of the Continuum.*
self-trust, 130, 135–136, 194
Set Your Mind (Rule of Disengagement), 148, 196
Setting Boundaries (Trait of Protective Offense), 60
Seven Rules of Disengagement. *see* Disengagement, Seven Rules of
sexual assault, 137, 148, 195, 204–205, 207, 210–211, 230, 235
sharp weapons, 156
Shooting the Gap, 193
silat, 244–245
silent interviews (MacYoung), 110–111
simplicity (in fighting), 191, 198
simulated self-defense encounters, 246–247
situational awareness, 9, 32, 59, 79–82, 101, 126, 149, 245, 251, 256
Situational Awareness, Active Listening, Intuition (Trait of Protective Offense), 59
sleep, healthy, 225–226, 231–233
slippery substances, as weapons, 157

slow practice, need for, 194, 198
social scripts, 34
social violence, 51–52, 53
sociopathy, 44–45, 47–49, 53
somatics, 227
split (positioning strategy), 126–127
stacking self-care modalities, 217, 231
Stand Your Ground laws, 195
stand-up grappling, 178
Stand-Your-Ground laws, 142–143
Stanley, Elizabeth, 228
stationary weapons, 157
STICC (shout, threaten, insult, challenge, command), 116
Stout, Martha, 47
Stout's Thirteen Rules, 47–49
strangers, teaching kids how to talk to, 254
stress, reframing, 20–22
strollers, maneuvering, 256
submission reaction, 144–145, 147
Sun Tzu, 39
surprise (positioning strategy), 125
surrounding (positioning strategy), 127, 192
sweeps, 171–172, 196
Systema, 247
Szal, Sara, 221
taekwondo, 247–248
tai chi chuan (taijiquan), 189, 223, 238, 248-249
team sports, 249
Ten Principles of Protective Offense, 267–269
therapy, 226–228
therapy pets, 218

threat displays, 88–89
threats of physical violence, 94
tonic immobility, 137
Triune Brain Theory, 23–25, 33
trust, misplaced, 97
tunnel vision, 145–146
Twelve Traits of Protective Offense, 57–65
undermining, 94
unfair fights, 134–135
van der Kolk, Bessel, 226, 228, 249
Verbal Communication (Trait of Protective Offense), 59–60
verbal deception, 92–93
Verbal Fence, 99–100, 103, 115
Viertl, Milan, 42–43
Violence Against Women Act, 211, 231
Visual Fence, 99–101, 103, 115
voice control, 59, 63
voice modulation, 59, 63
volunteering, 219
Vranich, Belisa, 224, 229
wanting, dangers of, 96–97
weapons, 153, 156–162, 196. *see also particular weapons*
weapons of opportunity, 161–162
Westen, Drew, 25
Wilder, Kris, 251
willingness and ability to fight, 137–141, 194
wushu, 246
xingyiquan, 189, 248–249
yoga, 255–256
Yousafzai, Malala, 141
Zombie Game, 256

Author Bio

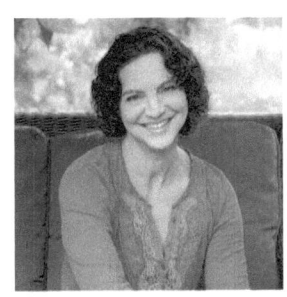

Tèja VanWicklen is a writer focused on reimagining self-defense for women and parents, and a consultant specializing in the depiction of realistic violence for fiction writers and filmmakers.

Teja has spent much of her life studying multiple martial arts, edged-weapons, firearms, wilderness survival, biomechanics, and health. She has seen martial arts and self-defense though many lenses: as a neglected, neurodivergent child raised around drugs and violence, an instructor, personal trainer, EMT, and manager of a stunt performance team. Teja has trained with elite military and law enforcement personnel and was a founding member of Conflict Research Group, a blog and information site run by a collective of renowned safety professionals. As manager of Art of War, Teja oversaw international stunt performances for major events, film festivals, and movie premieres worldwide, including the *Star Wars: Attack of the Clones* and *The Matrix: Reloaded* premiers in NYC and LA.

Teja has won grand championships, been featured in magazines, and interviewed for TV. Her screenplays have won awards and her short stories have been published in literary magazines (as Teja BenAmor).

Teja endured a difficult pregnancy and over a year of recuperation, which fundamentally changed her approach to self-defense and caused her to rethink her training. Her quest is to find the place where self-defense meets common sense; where self-awareness, situational awareness, strategy, and problem-solving intersect; to create a paradigm of empowerment for women who want to dismantle anxiety, see conflict as opportunity, and raise productive, resilient children who won't become victims (or criminals). *Reimagining Women's Self-Defense* is Teja's first book.

BOOKS FROM YMAA

- 101 REFLECTIONS ON TAI CHI CHUAN
- 108 INSIGHTS INTO TAI CHI CHUAN
- A WOMAN'S QIGONG GUIDE
- ADVANCING IN TAE KWON DO
- ANALYSIS OF GENUINE KARATE
- ANALYSIS OF GENUINE KARATE 2
- ANALYSIS OF SHU HA RI IN KARATE-DO
- ANALYSIS OF SHAOLIN CHIN NA 2ND ED
- ANCIENT CHINESE WEAPONS
- ART AND SCIENCE OF STAFF FIGHTING
- THE ART AND SCIENCE OF SELF-DEFENSE
- ART AND SCIENCE OF STICK FIGHTING
- ART OF HOJO UNDO
- ARTHRITIS RELIEF
- BACK PAIN RELIEF
- BAGUAZHANG
- BRAIN FITNESS
- CHIN NA IN GROUND FIGHTING
- CHINESE FAST WRESTLING
- CHINESE FITNESS
- CHINESE TUI NA MASSAGE
- COMPLETE MARTIAL ARTIST
- COMPREHENSIVE APPLICATIONS OF SHAOLIN CHIN NA
- CONFLICT COMMUNICATION
- DAO DE JING: A QIGONG INTERPRETATION
- DAO IN ACTION
- DEFENSIVE TACTICS
- DIRTY GROUND
- DR. WU'S HEAD MASSAGE
- ESSENCE OF SHAOLIN WHITE CRANE
- EXPLORING TAI CHI
- FACING VIOLENCE
- FIGHT LIKE A PHYSICIST
- THE FIGHTER'S BODY
- FIGHTER'S FACT BOOK 1&2
- FIGHTING THE PAIN RESISTANT ATTACKER
- FIRST DEFENSE
- FORCE DECISIONS: A CITIZENS GUIDE
- HOMECOMING SERIES
- INSIDE TAI CHI
- JUDO ADVANTAGE
- JUJI GATAME ENCYCLOPEDIA
- KARATE SCIENCE
- KEPPAN
- KRAV MAGA COMBATIVES
- KRAV MAGA FUNDAMENTAL STRATEGIES
- KRAV MAGA PROFESSIONAL TACTICS
- KRAV MAGA WEAPON DEFENSES
- LITTLE BLACK BOOK OF VIOLENCE
- LIUHEBAFA FIVE CHARACTER SECRETS
- MARTIAL ARTS OF VIETNAM
- MARTIAL ARTS INSTRUCTION
- MARTIAL WAY AND ITS VIRTUES
- MEDITATIONS ON VIOLENCE
- MERIDIAN QIGONG EXERCISES
- MINDFUL EXERCISE
- MIND INSIDE TAI CHI
- MIND INSIDE YANG STYLE TAI CHI CHUAN
- NORTHERN SHAOLIN SWORD
- OKINAWA'S COMPLETE KARATE SYSTEM: ISSHIN RYU
- PRINCIPLES OF TRADITIONAL CHINESE MEDICINE
- PROTECTOR ETHIC
- QIGONG FOR HEALTH & MARTIAL ARTS
- QIGONG FOR TREATING COMMON AILMENTS
- QIGONG MASSAGE
- QIGONG MEDITATION: EMBRYONIC BREATHING
- QIGONG GRAND CIRCULATION
- QIGONG MEDITATION: SMALL CIRCULATION
- QIGONG, THE SECRET OF YOUTH: DA MO'S CLASSICS
- ROOT OF CHINESE QIGONG
- SAFEST FAMILY ON THE BLOCK
- SAMBO ENCYCLOPEDIA
- SCALING FORCE
- SELF-DEFENSE FOR WOMEN
- SHIN GI TAI: KARATE TRAINING
- SIMPLE CHINESE MEDICINE
- SIMPLE QIGONG EXERCISES FOR HEALTH, 3RD ED.
- SIMPLIFIED TAI CHI CHUAN, 2ND ED.
- SOLO TRAINING 1&2
- SPOTTING DANGER BEFORE IT SPOTS YOU
- SPOTTING DANGER BEFORE IT SPOTS YOUR KIDS
- SPOTTING DANGER BEFORE IT SPOTS YOUR TEENS
- SPOTTING DANGER FOR TRAVELERS
- SUMO FOR MIXED MARTIAL ARTS
- SUNRISE TAI CHI
- SURVIVING ARMED ASSAULTS
- TAE KWON DO: THE KOREAN MARTIAL ART
- TAEKWONDO BLACK BELT POOMSAE
- TAEKWONDO: A PATH TO EXCELLENCE
- TAEKWONDO: ANCIENT WISDOM
- TAEKWONDO: DEFENSE AGAINST WEAPONS
- TAEKWONDO: SPIRIT AND PRACTICE
- TAI CHI BALL QIGONG: FOR HEALTH AND MARTIAL ARTS
- TAI CHI BALL QIGONG
- THE TAI CHI BOOK
- TAI CHI CHIN NA
- TAI CHI CHUAN CLASSICAL YANG STYLE
- TAI CHI CHUAN MARTIAL APPLICATIONS
- TAI CHI CHUAN MARTIAL POWER
- TAI CHI CONCEPTS AND EXPERIMENTS
- TAI CHI DYNAMICS
- TAI CHI FOR DEPRESSION
- TAI CHI IN 10 WEEKS
- TAI CHI PUSH HANDS
- TAI CHI QIGONG
- TAI CHI SECRETS OF THE ANCIENT MASTERS
- TAI CHI SECRETS OF THE WU & LI STYLES
- TAI CHI SECRETS OF THE WU STYLE
- TAI CHI SECRETS OF THE YANG STYLE
- TAI CHI SWORD: CLASSICAL YANG STYLE
- TAI CHI SWORD FOR BEGINNERS
- TAI CHI WALKING
- TAI CHI CHUAN THEORY OF DR. YANG, JWING-MING
- TOP TEN KICKS
- FIGHTING ARTS
- TRADITIONAL CHINESE HEALTH SECRETS
- TRADITIONAL TAEKWONDO
- TRAINING FOR SUDDEN VIOLENCE
- TRIANGLE HOLD ENCYCLOPEDIA
- TRUE WELLNESS SERIES (MIND, HEART, GUT)
- WARRIOR'S MANIFESTO
- WAY OF KATA
- WAY OF SANCHIN KATA
- WAY TO BLACK BELT
- WESTERN HERBS FOR MARTIAL ARTISTS
- WILD GOOSE QIGONG
- WING CHUN IN-DEPTH
- WINNING FIGHTS
- XINGYIQUAN

AND MANY MORE . . .

VIDEOS FROM YMAA

- ANALYSIS OF SHAOLIN CHIN NA
- ART AND SCIENCE OF SELF DEFENSE
- ART AND SCIENCE OF STAFF FIGHTING
- ART AND SCIENCE STICK FIGHTING
- ART AND SCIENCE SWORD FIGHTING
- BAGUA FOR BEGINNERS 1 & 2
- BEGINNER QIGONG FOR WOMEN 1 & 2
- BEGINNER TAI CHI FOR HEALTH
- BREATH MEDICINE
- BIOENERGY TRAINING 1&2
- CHEN TAI CHI CANNON FIST
- CHEN TAI CHI FIRST FORM
- CHEN TAI CHI FOR BEGINNERS
- CHIN NA IN-DEPTH SERIES
- FACING VIOLENCE: 7 THINGS A MARTIAL ARTIST MUST KNOW
- FIVE ANIMAL SPORTS
- FIVE ELEMENTS ENERGY BALANCE
- HEALER WITHIN: MEDICAL QIGONG
- INFIGHTING
- INTRODUCTION TO QI GONG FOR BEGINNERS
- JOINT LOCKS
- KUNG FU BODY CONDITIONING 1 & 2
- KUNG FU FOR KIDS AND TEENS SERIES
- MERIDIAN QIGONG
- NEIGONG FOR MARTIAL ARTS
- NORTHERN SHAOLIN SWORD
- QI GONG 30-DAY CHALLENGE
- QI GONG FOR ANXIETY
- QI GONG FOR ARMS, WRISTS, AND HANDS
- QIGONG FOR BEGINNERS: FRAGRANCE
- QI GONG FOR BETTER BALANCE
- QI GONG FOR BETTER BREATHING
- QI GONG FOR CANCER
- QI GONG FOR DEPRESSION
- QI GONG FOR ENERGY AND VITALITY
- QI GONG FOR HEADACHES
- QIGONG FOR HEALTH: BETTER DIGESTION
- QIGONG FOR HEALTH: HEALING QIGONG EXERCISES
- QIGONG FOR HEALTH: IMMUNE SYSTEM
- QIGONG FOR HEALTH: JOINT REHABILITATION
- QIGONG FOR HEALTH: MERIDIAN EXTREMITIES
- QIGONG FOR HEALTH: SITTING QIGONG EXERCISES
- QIGONG FOR HEALTH: SPINE AND BACK
- QI GONG FOR THE HEALTHY HEART
- QI GONG FOR HEALTHY JOINTS
- QI GONG FOR HIGH BLOOD PRESSURE
- QIGONG FOR LONGEVITY
- QI GONG FOR STRONG BONES
- QI GONG FOR THE UPPER BACK AND NECK
- QIGONG FOR WOMEN WITH DAISY LEE
- QIGONG FLOW FOR STRESS & ANXIETY RELIEF
- QIGONG GRAND CIRCULATION
- QIGONG MASSAGE
- QIGONG MINDFULNESS IN MOTION
- QI GONG—THE SEATED WORKOUT
- QIGONG: 15 MINUTES TO HEALTH
- SABER FUNDAMENTAL TRAINING
- SAI TRAINING AND SEQUENCES
- SANCHIN KATA: TRADITIONAL TRAINING FOR KARATE POWER
- SCALING FORCE
- SEARCHING FOR SUPERHUMANS
- SHAOLIN KUNG FU FUNDAMENTAL TRAINING: COURSES 1 & 2
- SHAOLIN LONG FIST KUNG FU BEGINNER-INTERMEDIATE-ADVANCED SERIES
- SHAOLIN SABER: BASIC SEQUENCES
- SHAOLIN STAFF: BASIC SEQUENCES
- SHAOLIN WHITE CRANE GONG FU BASIC TRAINING SERIES
- SHUAI JIAO: KUNG FU WRESTLING
- SIMPLE QIGONG EXERCISES FOR HEALTH
- SIMPLE QIGONG EXERCISES FOR ARTHRITIS RELIEF
- SIMPLE QIGONG EXERCISES FOR BACK PAIN RELIEF
- SIMPLIFIED TAI CHI CHUAN: 24 & 48 POSTURES
- SIMPLIFIED TAI CHI FOR BEGINNERS 48
- SPOTTING DANGER BEFORE IT SPOTS YOU
- SPOTTING DANGER FOR KIDS
- SPOTTING DANGER FOR TEENS
- SUN TAI CHI
- SWORD: FUNDAMENTAL TRAINING
- TAEKWONDO KORYO POOMSAE
- TAI CHI BALL QIGONG SERIES
- TAI CHI BALL WORKOUT FOR BEGINNERS
- TAI CHI CHUAN CLASSICAL YANG STYLE
- TAI CHI FIGHTING SET
- TAI CHI FIT: 24 FORM
- TAI CHI FIT: ALZHEIMER'S PREVENTION
- TAI CHI FIT: CANCER PREVENTION
- TAI CHI FIT FOR VETERANS
- TAI CHI FIT: FOR WOMEN
- TAI CHI FIT: FLOW
- TAI CHI FIT: FUSION BAMBOO
- TAI CHI FIT: FUSION FIRE
- TAI CHI FIT: FUSION IRON
- TAI CHI FIT: HEALTHY BACK SEATED WORKOUT
- TAI CHI FIT: HEALTHY HEART WORKOUT
- TAI CHI FIT IN PARADISE
- TAI CHI FIT: OVER 50
- TAI CHI FIT OVER 50: BALANCE EXERCISES
- TAI CHI FIT OVER 50: SEATED WORKOUT
- TAI CHI FIT OVER 60: GENTLE EXERCISES
- TAI CHI FIT OVER 60: HEALTHY JOINTS
- TAI CHI FIT OVER 60: LIVE LONGER
- TAI CHI FIT: STRENGTH
- TAI CHI FIT: TO GO
- TAI CHI FOR WOMEN
- TAI CHI FUSION: FIRE
- TAI CHI QIGONG
- TAI CHI PRINCIPLES FOR HEALTHY AGING
- TAI CHI PUSHING HANDS SERIES
- TAI CHI SWORD: CLASSICAL YANG STYLE
- TAI CHI SWORD FOR BEGINNERS
- TAI CHI SYMBOL: YIN YANG STICKING HANDS
- TAIJI & SHAOLIN STAFF: FUNDAMENTAL TRAINING
- TAIJI CHIN NA IN-DEPTH
- TAIJI 37 POSTURES MARTIAL APPLICATIONS
- TAIJI SABER CLASSICAL YANG STYLE
- TAIJI WRESTLING
- TRAINING FOR SUDDEN VIOLENCE
- UNDERSTANDING QIGONG SERIES
- WHITE CRANE HARD & SOFT QIGONG
- YANG TAI CHI FOR BEGINNERS
- YOQI: MICROCOSMIC ORBIT QIGONG
- YOQI QIGONG FOR A HAPPY HEART
- YOQI:QIGONG FLOW FOR HAPPY MIND
- YOQI:QIGONG FLOW FOR INTERNAL ALCHEMY
- YOQI QIGONG FOR HAPPY SPLEEN & STOMACH
- YOQI QIGONG FOR HAPPY KIDNEYS
- YOQI QIGONG FLOW FOR HAPPY LUNGS
- YOQI QIGONG FLOW FOR STRESS RELIEF
- YOQI: QIGONG FLOW TO BOOST IMMUNE SYSTEM
- YOQI SIX HEALING SOUNDS
- YOQI: YIN YOGA 1
- WU TAI CHI FOR BEGINNERS
- WUDANG KUNG FU: FUNDAMENTAL TRAINING
- WUDANG SWORD
- WUDANG TAIJIQUAN
- XINGYIQUAN
- YANG TAI CHI FOR BEGINNERS

AND MANY MORE . . .

more products available from . . .

YMAA Publication Center, Inc.   楊氏東方文化出版中心

1-800-669-8892 • info@ymaa.com • www.ymaa.com

www.ingramcontent.com/pod-product-compliance
Lightning Source LLC
Chambersburg PA
CBHW030511080526
44586CB00011B/143